Aromatic Waters: Therapeutic, Cosmetic, and Culinary Hydrosol Applications

AMY KREYDIN

INTRODUCTION

I grew up in Questa, a village in the lower Rockies nestled into the Sangre de Cristo mountains in northern New Mexico. My mother taught me how to garden and inspired my lifelong love of plants, and my father taught me how to work with wood to build furniture, goat sheds, and homes. Summers found me apprenticed to farmers with greenhouses, midwives at the birth center in Taos, wildcrafting herbs with the village curandera, bundling Artemisia tridentata into incense sticks for the flea market in Santa Fe, making fruit leathers in Dede's adobe kitchen, or building a sweat lodge. It was a weird and wonderful childhood in one of my favorite places on the planet.

This foundation put me on the path of studying botanical medicine and the healing arts for the better part of two decades. In 2004 I opened my private practice, The Barefoot Dragonfly, offering my services as a newly certified Foot, Hand, and Ear Reflexologist, a modality which employs finger and pressure techniques applied to maps that resemble the human body. Five years later, in 2009, I jumped at the opportunity to study essential oils in the evidence-based *Clinical Aromatherapy for Health Professionals* course with Kathy Duffy, at one of the Harvard teaching hospitals in Boston. A year later, I had my 250-hour *Certified Clinical Aromatherapy Practitioner*, or CCAP. Since then, my education in the therapeutic, culinary, and cosmetic applications of essential oils, hydrosols, absolutes, and carbon dioxide extracts, has grown.

Hydrosols make their way into culinary dishes and beverages in my kitchen, and into cosmetic and therapeutic formulations in my studio. I distill a number of plants and herbs from my apothecary garden, and I teach a four-week introductory course on hydrosols as part of my 200-hour Professional Aromatherapy Certification program.

The Barefoot Dragonfly is the name of my business and I offer private sessions and consultations as well as educational courses and classes. I advocate for consumers to make informed decisions about their wellness care by presenting evidence-based information on botanicals, through a lens of Eastern medicine. No two people on this planet will present with the exact same wellness challenges and their remedies therefore cannot be identical. I hope this book acts as a guide as you start or expand your knowledge of hydrosols and holistic medicine.

In health,

Amy Kreydin, NBCR, CCAP, BD
Board Certified Reflexologist
Clinical Aromatherapy Practitioner
Aromatic Medicine Practitioner
Metamorphic Technique Practitioner
DONA Trained Birth Doula

AMY KREYDIN

CONTENTS

PART I: UNDERSTANDING HYDROSOLS

1 WHAT IS A HYDROSOL?

A hydrosol is the water distillate formed in the process of steam and/or water distillation. Specifically, in the aromatherapy community, we use the term *hydrosol* to define the water distillate formed from botanical material that is distilled. An understanding of the process of distillation will help to better define a true hydrosol:

- The person distilling will load the still with fresh water and botanical material.
- The still is placed on a heating element, causing the water to boil and transform into steam.
- The steam then travels up through the plant matter, capturing the plant's cellular water and volatile oils (essential oils), as it travels.
- The steam reaches the end of its path at a dual-chambered tube, called the condensing coil.
- On the outside of the coil, the distiller uses a pump to run chilled water over the coil.
- Once the steam reaches the inside of the coil, it is rapidly cooled and transforms from its vapour state back into its liquid state, water.
- The distiller collects this liquid and skims or filters any visible essential oils into a separate vessel.

The end result in this production is an aromatic water that is approximately 20-30 times stronger than an herbal tea and has roughly 0.02%-0.05% volatile oils (Chemistry of hydrosols: What's in the waters? A. Harman, 2015). These micro-particles of volatile oils are so small that they cannot be observed by the naked eye, but they can be detected using lab equipment such as *gas chromatography/mass spectrometry* (GCMS) and *solid phase microextraction (SPME)*.

Hydrosol, Hydrolat, Aromatic Water – What's in a Name?

In what has proven to be a teaching and marketing headache for many of us in the aromatherapy community, our beloved aqueous solution has gone by a number of different names.

Here are some of the more common ones in circulation today:

- **Hydrosol** - a pairing of the Greek word for water (*hydro*) and the Latin word *solver* which means to loosen or solve. This term is my favorite because it represents a water solvent, an apt description of our water distillate.
- **Hydrolat** – the French observed that some hydrosols initially come out of the still looking every bit like a glass of watery milk (Faucon 2012). So hydro stayed but *lait,* meaning milk in French, was added. A lot of aromatherapists still use this term, but the phenomenon in which the distillate is milky resolves into a clear liquid within hours, days, or weeks, so by the time the consumer has it in hand, it isn't actually a glass of watery milk, or hydrolat, any longer.
- **Aromatic Water** – I've found this term a bit easier to use around the uninitiated, but it isn't wholly accurate, since some hydrosols produced have very little aroma to them. For example, calendula and echinacea hydrosols are very low-odor and smell a bit like a boring herbal tea. When compared with a bright aroma like rose hydrosol, they are a bit disappointing to the nose.
- **Essential Waters or Essential Oil Waters** – this is another term that attempts to present this solution to a novice, but isn't completely accurate either, as some hydrosols are distilled from plants that have no volatile oils in them at all.
- **Floral Waters** – who wouldn't want a floral water on their vanity? But what about the floral waters not distilled from actual flowers, like the bright lemongrass hydrosol distilled from the leaves of the lemongrass plant or the crisp pine hydrosol distilled from the needles or cones or bark of the pine tree? A lovely name, but it falls short in defining the breadth of hydrosols available to us.

For the sake of organization and clarity, I will be using the term "hydrosol" throughout this book. If in your mind you replace that term with something that suits your learning experience better, I welcome the creativity!

What Do Folks Do with Hydrosols?

Hydrosols smell a bit like their essential oil cousins, but they aren't as popular outside of the aromatherapy profession. When I was first introduced to hydrosols, I loved using them as face spritzers to moisten my skin before applying a lotion or cream in the mornings and evenings. Later, I thought I'd invented the idea of using them in the hair during cold winters in New England, when low humidity can cause a perfectly good head of hair to become some kind of poltergeist. Over the years, I've learned from other aromatherapists, artisan distillers, and herbalists how they use hydrosols. The uses I will cover in this book include:

- Cosmetic – hydrating, toning, and nourishing the integumentary system
- Therapeutic – allies in wellness plans from acute to chronic imbalances
- Culinary – flavor and aroma enhancers for foods and beverages

Hydrosols have a long history of use, but up until recently they were primarily used to impart flavor for medicines, or used as a fragrance for cosmetics. You'll see these two uses are still applicable today; we've just discovered that they have so many more uses!

2 WHAT TO LOOK FOR IN A QUALITY HYDROSOL

Anytime a health-supporting product gains popularity, we see a matching rise in cheaply produced products flooding the market. Unfortunately, this is only too true with hydrosols. The real concern is the risk of an unwanted outcome when an inferior product is used. I'm starting to hear of weeks-long illnesses from contaminated or fake hydrosols, and that makes me sad and frustrated.

When looking for authentic hydrosols, we want a product that has been distilled expressly for the purposes of getting a hydrosol. The leftover biowaste from distilling essential oils isn't considered an authentic hydrosol (but that doesn't prevent it from frequently being sold as such). Steps that a distiller needs to consider when producing hydrosols include water quality, freshness of plant material, sterilization of equipment, hygiene control for all members of the distilling and bottling crew, and appropriate storage conditions following distillation. The initial costs present a hurdle to a distiller who will have to reeducate employees, and may have to install cold storage facilities if he/she is in a hot climate.

What I look for in the production and storage of a quality hydrosol:

- **Fresh plant material** – unlike essential oil distillation, where plants are partially dried prior to being loaded into a still, we want the cellular water in fresh, unwilted plants for hydrosols. There is an exception here for plants that don't have abundant cellular water – resins, barks, and seeds are good examples of botanical materials that need a good soak in water prior to distilling them.
- **Pure water** – the goals here are, one, to avoid waters treated with chemicals and, two, to have the highest quality water in this product. Remember that a hydrosol is 99+% water, so the better the water, the better the hydrosol. My colleagues who distill use purified water from natural springs, aquifers, lakes, and rainwater in their hydrosol distillations.
- **Sanitation and Good Manufacturing Practices** – hydrosols are highly susceptible to deterioration through contamination, as they are not routinely preserved. The distiller and retailer/rebottler should be employing what is known as current good manufacturing practices, or cGMP, in order to maintain the purity of the hydrosol. Steps should be taken to sterilize all vessels the

hydrosol comes into contact with, and a clean room should be used when transferring from large drums and jugs into smaller bottles for retail.

- **Preservative-Free** – this might seem like a bad idea, I mean, who wants something that could spoil quickly? Hear me out though. A hydrosol that has been adulterated with preservatives may not be safe to use in the kitchen, on the skin, or by mouth. Which rules out all of the uses I recommend in this book.
- **Cold storage** – unpreserved hydrosols need to be stored in cool conditions to ensure that their shelf-life is stable. Cold storage may mean refrigeration or in a root or wine cellar. If a hydrosol is sitting on the shelves at the indie or big box health food store, keep on walking.

How will you know if the distiller and retailer have followed these guidelines? You'll have to ask!

3 QUESTIONS TO ASK TO DETERMINE QUALITY AND SAFETY OF A HYDROSOL

For safety reasons, we want to be concerned about contaminated, adulterated, and improperly stored hydrosols before we use them. Here are some of the questions I like to ask before considering a hydrosol purchase from a new-to-me distiller or retailer:

- What is the binomial (Latin) name of the plant that this aromatic extract comes from?
- Does it have a chemotype? (e.g., Rosemary Ct Cineole)
- How was the plant grown?
- Was this distilled for the hydrosol or is this biowaste from distilling an essential oil?
- What type of still was used? (e.g., glass, stainless steel, copper)
- When was it distilled (month and year) and what have been the storage conditions since?
- Is this hydrosol preserved?
- Have any other additives been used in this hydrosol? (e.g., colorants, solubolizers, stabilizers)
- What microbiological testing has been done? Can I have a copy of the test results?
- Do you rebottle the hydrosol from barrels into smaller bottles? Is this done in a clean room that meets current good manufacturing practices (cGMP)?

There are very real concerns of being poisoned by adulterants and being infected by contaminants in hydrosols. If you're unsure if a hydrosol is safe to use around the mucous membranes, orally, or on the skin, it is better not to use it than to risk an unwanted outcome.

Of importance: once a hydrosol has spoiled it cannot be used safely. Store your hydrosols in clear containers and check it before each use for signs of spoilage: little specs floating in the bottom of the bottle up to large fungal blooms in the middle. If you're distilling your own hydrosols and not keeping cGMP practices and rebottling in a clean room, it would be prudent to run a water analysis test for bacteria, and fungi routinely throughout the life of the hydrosol.

4 A NOTE ON COPPER STILLS

Copper stills are quite *en vogue* for hydrosol distillation at the moment, and for a good reason – they appear to extend the shelf-life of a hydrosol. When botanical materials are distilled in a copper vessel, some of the copper is taken up in the steam and comes over into the water. (Harman 2012). While technically this is a contamination of the hydrosol, it is thought to be a useful contamination because of its capacity to extend the shelf-life of the hydrosol itself. Studies have found that when copper is used on touch surfaces like hospital door handles and bedrails, it neutralizes microbes, and is therefore considered an antimicrobial agent (Grass, Rensing, Solioz 2011).

On the flip side are the concerns around copper distillates in oral dosing, and these concerns warrant additional research. A couple of my concerns are for those diagnosed with thyroid disorders, as copper has a thyroid down-regulating effect (Iseki, Atsushi, et al 2000), and has a competitive relationship with zinc absorption (Oestreicher, Cousins 1985), which may serve to exacerbate hypothyroidism and Hashimoto's disease.

Another concern with copper distillates is in the population with known and unknown metal hypersensitivities. Those of us who know we're allergic to metals like copper tend to avoid drinking out of copper cups, imbibing whiskey regularly or at all, and consuming copper-distilled hydrosols. For me, when I do any of these, I get variations of a slight oral reaction, which usually means my tongue and mouth feel funny. Clients that have had negative reactions to copper-distilled hydrosols report rashes on the neck and/or torso, nausea, headaches, and joint pain. It usually takes daily oral or dermal application before symptoms arise, but I've had a few clients with severe multiple chemical sensitivities (MCS) that have reacted after a single application. If you suspect a copper allergy/sensitivity, you can try doing a copper patch test in which you walk around with a piece of copper, like a penny, taped to your forearm for 48-hours. You can also see what your options are for metal allergy testing with your local allergist. Or you can avoid copper-distilled hydrosols altogether.

5 THERAPEUTIC USE OF HYDROSOLS

Hydrosols can be employed in health and wellness plans to support the mind, body, and spirit. They do a lovely job of it and I hope this introduction to, or extension of education in, hydrosols inspires you to make friends with these plant allies of ours.

Within the framework of the holistic modality of aromatherapy, hydrosols can be used on their own, as is, or in formulations with other botanical ingredients. For the purposes of brevity, we'll be exploring just hydrosols as the sole active ingredient in this chapter. When we get to the hydrosol monographs, you'll see recipes and formulations that expand the knowledge base you acquire in this chapter and give you some room to play and explore.

Please note that I prefer to use the metric system of measurements for hydrosols, as it gives a more reliable way of dosing. For readers who are used to the imperial system of measurements, a great hack for this would be to pick up one of those shot glass-sized measuring glasses at the local culinary specialty shop or the kitchenware department of most big box stores. These wee glasses look like a standard shot glass, but have demarcations on the side noting volume in milliliters, teaspoons, tablespoons, and ounces. They're brilliant and can survive dozens of washings in the dishwasher before the lines fade.

Oral Dosing

If you'll recall from the *What Is a Hydrosol?* chapter, a hydrosol is roughly 20-30 times stronger than an herbal tea. When adding a hydrosol to a glass of juice, water, or tea, it doesn't need a dispersing agent like an essential oil would, as the essential oil constituents in the hydrosol are already evenly dispersed.

Determining how much hydrosol to use in an oral dose depends on the therapeutic goals and the length of use planned. **For adults** consider these guidelines:

Health maintenance: 5-15 ml (1 teaspoon to 1 tablespoon) hydrosol to 4-6 ounces purified water, juice, or tea, taken twice a day. This lower dose would be for long-term support of the endocrine, digestive, and/or nervous systems of the body. Think menopause, indigestion or constipation, chronic insomnia, alongside treatment for anxiety or depression, and premenstrual syndrome (PMS).

Acute health support: 30-45 ml (2-3 tablespoons) to 4-6 ounces purified water, juice, or tea, taken twice a day. This higher dose would be for short-term support of the endocrine, digestive, and/or nervous systems of the body. Think travel-induced nausea, pain management after straining muscles painting the kitchen or doing yard work, flatulence, acute stressors like pre-wedding jitters or a pending exam, and short-term insomnia around the full moon or after changing time zones.

For children I usually find that adding the hydrosol to juice makes it more palatable, though I avoid this practice in very young children. For children 2 years of age and younger, you can dilute juice in water using 1 part juice to 10 parts water, or 1 ounce juice to 10 ounces water. You can then add the hydrosol to however many ounces of the diluted juice you are going to use and refrigerate the rest for later.

Pediatric Dose Guidelines:
- **Newborns to 6 months**: Oral use of hydrosols can interfere with breast and bottle feeding, so I generally reserve this intervention for acute cases of infection under the guidance of a practitioner with experience in this area.
- **6-12 months**: 5 ml (1 teaspoon) to 8 ounces purified water or juice and served in 2-4 ounce increments throughout the day.
- **1-9 years**: 10 ml (2 teaspoons) to 4 ounces purified water, tea, or juice, once or twice a day.
- **10-14 years**: 20-30 mls (4 teaspoons to 2 tablespoons) to 4 ounces purified water, tea, or juice, once or twice a day.

Dermal Dosing

Hydrosols don't have to be diluted for adults. They can applied directly to the skin via a spritz bottle, a small cloth or cotton round soaked in the hydrosol, or in a small basin to soak a region of the skin like the hands or feet. There's no harm in diluting for adults though, especially if you have sensitive skin or simply want your hydrosol to last longer.

Guidelines for diluting hydrosols for children:

- **Newborns to 6 months**: 1:4 – 1 part hydrosol to 4 parts purified water.
- **6 months to 2 years**: 1:2 – 1 part hydrosol to 2 parts purified water.
- **2 years and older**: 1:1 – 1 part hydrosol to 1 part purified water.

Direct Inhalation

My aromatic medicine instructor, Mark Webb, introduced me to direct inhalation of hydrosols with equal parts of rose and rosemary hydrosols. Oh my goodness was that divine! My shoulders came down from supporting my earlobes, and my eyes rolled into the back of my head. Wow!

I use a handheld nebulizer I got from Amazon for less than $30 from a company called Uniclife. I sterilize the unit with an alcohol-based cleaning spray to prepare it for use. Then, I fill the basin with 25 mls (5 teaspoons) distilled or purified water (I don't use tap water for the risk of fungal contaminants being driven into the airways), and add up to 10 mls (2 teaspoons) of my hydrosol(s) of choice to the dosing cup provided. I place the adult or pediatric mask on the machine, plug it in, and give a ten-minute inhaled dose.

I recommend this method to students and clients for:
- sinus congestion
- cough and sore throat
- dry airways from visits to the mountains or desert
- before and after stage performance for voice actors and singers
- prior to meditating or a yoga practice
- following a massage, reflexology, or acupuncture treatment
- before and after talk therapy

Nebulizers can dose the respiratory system with hydrosols and be used at full strength for adults and children 10 years and older. For younger children dilute 1:4 or 1:2. I do not recommend adding essential oils unless you disperse them in the hydrosol with a solubilizing agent. I also recommend not exceeding the 10-minute dosing for adults or children, as there is a risk of ciliostasis, a condition in which the hair-like follicles in the lungs cease to move, causing fluid to collect instead of being expelled.

Indirect Inhalation

Hydrosols can be added to the basin of many essential oil diffusers – look for the types of diffusers that normally have a basin of water, and add 5-15 mls (1-3 teaspoons) of your hydrosol(s).

A spritz bottle can also be used as a room spray filled with 25-100% hydrosol(s) and sprayed high into a room, or over fabrics (test an inconspicuous area to be sure it won't stain) like bed linens or curtains to passively diffuse a room. I'm fond of lavender and marjoram hydrosol spritzed on my pillowcase prior to sleep, and lemon or cedarwood hydrosol spritzed in the linen closet or drawers to freshen fabrics.

PART II: HYDROSOL PROFILES

6 MONOGRAPHS

The following monographs include my clinical and personal experiences with a number of my favorite hydrosols.

Each monograph gives you a brief background on the botanical, its common name(s) as well as botanical name(s), and what botanical family it comes from (e.g., Lamiaceae, Verbenaceae). The text also presents the parts of the plant generally used to produce the hydrosol, a description of the odor of the hydrosol, and, when applicable, its flavor. When available, any safety considerations attributed to the plant, hydrosol, or essential oil are noted. I also include biophysical actions, some usage suggestions, and, when available, a culinary, cosmetic, or therapeutic recipe to try at home.

The biophysical actions I attribute to hydrosols in this book are mainly based on my first-hand experiences and not on current research data. Hydrosols haven't had the level of research and historical usage that their herb and essential oil counterparts have had. I think with their rise in popularity, we will see more research done on authentic hydrosols via universities around the globe. Disappointingly, many of the studies you might find with a casual scholar.google.com search are done using biowaste waters from distilling essential oils.

Until we have better access to studies, I hope this information helps you in your explorations, gives you some guidelines, and inspires you to undertake some independent experiences yourself on what an individual hydrosol can offer for your wellness plans. I'd love to hear about your experiences, recipes, and formulations at info@thebarefootdragonfly.com.

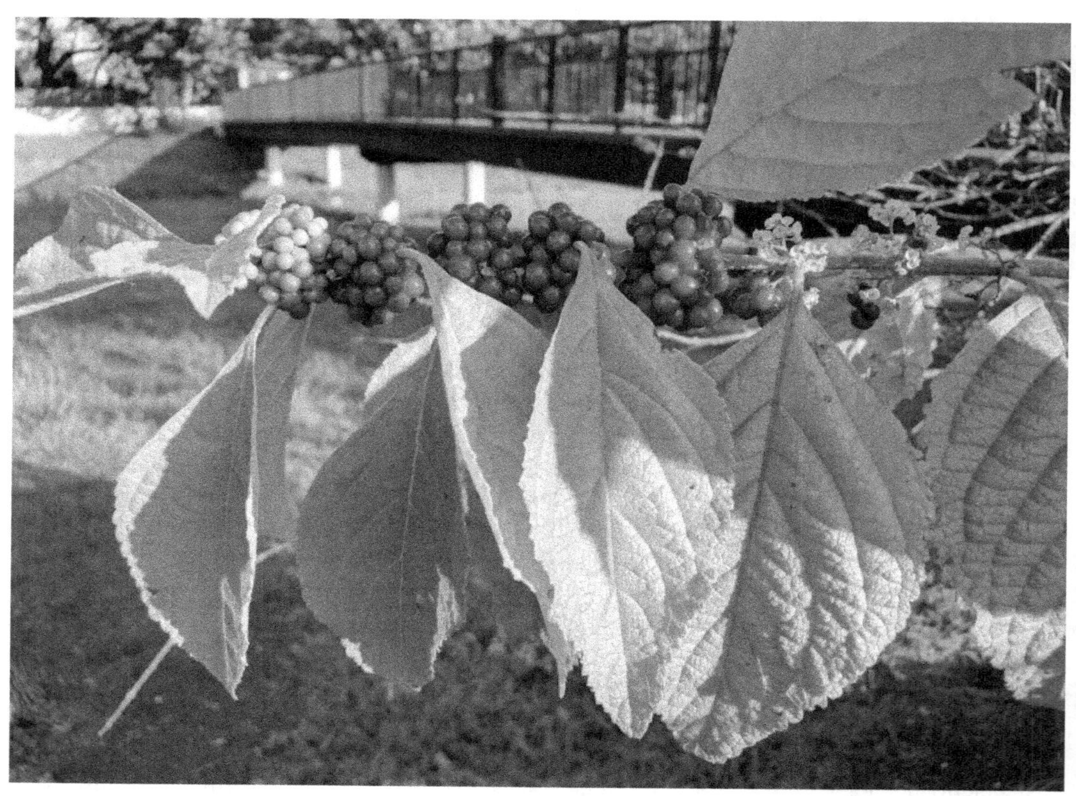

7 AMERICAN BEAUTYBERRY

The American Beautyberry is known for its showy, jewel-toned berries produced in the summer to early fall. It grows in the Southeastern to South Central region of the United States from Maryland to Texas.

In the early 1900s, farmers would crush the leaves of the beautyberry bush and rub themselves and their livestock down to repel mosquitoes and biting insects (Brakie 2010). Today, the hydrosol is used in bug sprays to repel mosquitoes -- and I've had success using it to repel our infamous Texas fire ant from the walkways and porch areas, when liberally sprayed.

Common Name(s): American Beautyberry
Botanical Name(s): *Callicarpa americana L.*
Botanical Family: Verbenaceae – Verbena family
Plant Parts Used: Leaves
Odor Profile: Light green scent
Flavor: Not for internal use
Safety Considerations: For external use only
Biophysical Actions: insect repellent

Bug Spray

2 ounces beautyberry hydrosol
1 ounce basil hydrosol
180 mg xanthan gum
270 mg glucanolactone and sodium benzoate (GSB)
5 drops lemon tea tree essential oil
8 drops catnip essential oil
10 drops patchouli essential oil
31 drops palmarosa essential oil

Heat the hydrosol to lukewarm and add it to a small bowl. Sprinkle the xanthan gum powder and the GSB over the surface and let sit for a couple minutes. Whisk ingredients together for a minute and let sit again for several minutes. Whisk once more then transfer to a 3-ounce bottle with a spray nozzle. Add essential oils, and shake well to disperse.

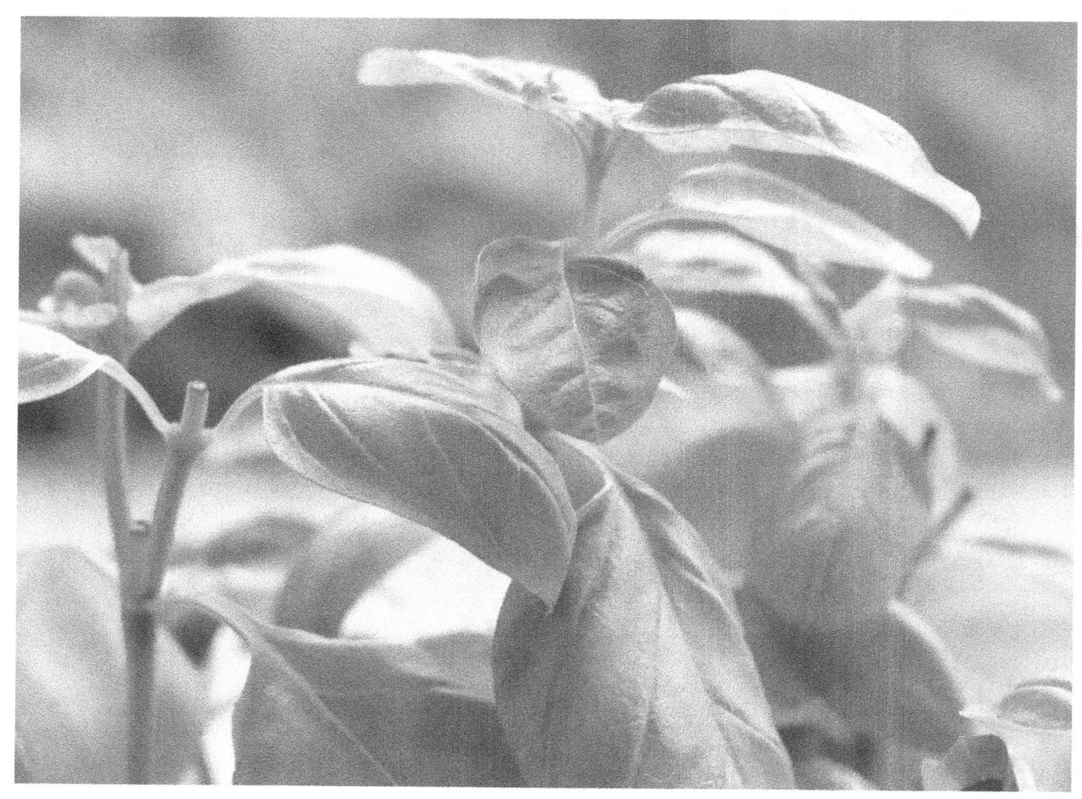

8 BASIL, SWEET

Basil has a number of different species and the basilicum variety has different chemotypes. A basil hydrosol that has a bit of a licorice aroma to it is going to be higher in eugenol, which has some safety considerations and is recommended to avoid during pregnancy, breastfeeding, and by young children.

Basil is a very common culinary herb and the essential oil has a history of use as an antifungal, mosquito repellent, insect repellent, and a mental stimulant.

Common Name(s): Sweet Basil, French Basil, Common Basil, Tropical Basil, Exotic Basil
Botanical Name(s): *Ocimum basilicum*
Botanical Family: Lamiaceae – Mint Family
Plant Parts Used: Leaves and flowers

Odor Profile: Rich floral-basil aroma
Flavor: Pungent, peppery, mildly floral
Safety Considerations: It may be prudent to restrict usage of hydrosols distilled from botanicals known for their high eugenol and estragole content during pregnancy, breastfeeding, in pediatrics, and those with ulcers or clotting disorders, until further research can be done to assess risk
Biophysical Actions: emotionally uplifting, insect and mosquito repellent, mental restorative

Basil hydrosol smells like a bowl of pesto with a bit of a floral nose to it. If you're fond of pesto like I am, then you'll delight in the aroma of this hydrosol! I love adding a teaspoon to my spaghetti sauce right before serving, a splash in gazpacho soup, and a spritz to my peach shrub cocktail for a tropical, spicy nose. This hydrosol also makes its way into bug sprays and I love it co-distilled with lemongrass to pep up my Thai peanut sauce.

In addition to all of these fun culinary uses, I love to use this hydrosol when I'm ready to switch gears – e.g., when I'm ready to transition from small business owner, doing SOAP notes or preparing taxes, to playtime mode, when I'm ready to go paddleboarding or enjoy a night on the town with friends. I use this in either a glass of water or I'll spritz my face and décolletage.

Cold Zucchini Soup

This soup is one of my favorites to bring out at the first sign of zucchini season in the garden!

2 tablespoons olive oil
1 tablespoon unsalted butter
1 garlic clove, minced
2 onions, finely chopped
2-3 large or 4-6 small zucchini, small diced
6 cups stock, chicken or vegetable
1 ounce basil hydrosol
1 tablespoon fresh lemon juice
Freshly ground black pepper

Place the diced zucchini in a colander and salt them. Sauté garlic and onion in butter and olive oil. Add zucchini and cook for a few minutes to soften. Then add stock and bring to a simmer. Cook until zucchini is fork-tender, remove from heat, and then blend with an immersion blender until smooth. Stir in the hydrosol, lemon juice, and season with salt and pepper. Chill until it has reached desired temperature. Serve.

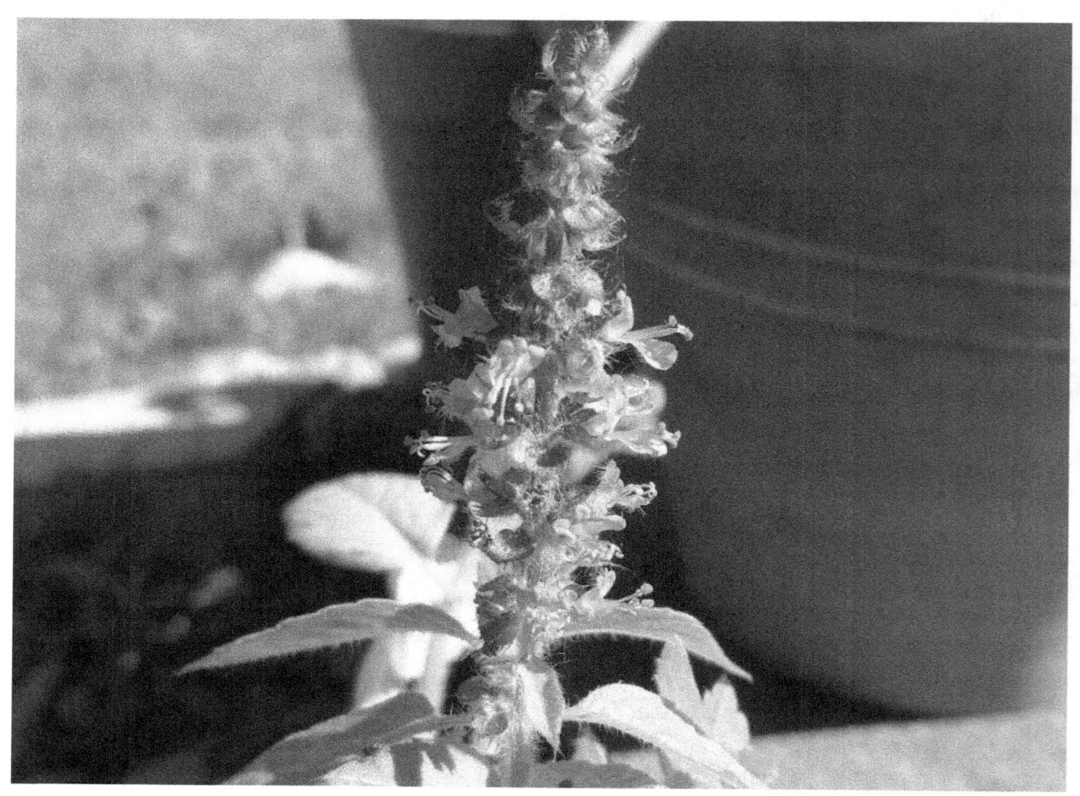

9 BASIL, HOLY

Holy Basil, also known as Tulsi, is indigenous to India, parts of North and Eastern Africa, Taiwan, and China. This herb grows up to 1 meter (3 feet) in height, with attractive green leaves that are smaller and more oblong than the basilicum basil.

Tulsi is considered a sacred plant in Hindu homes, where it is worshipped as the reincarnation of the goddess *Tulsi Vrindavan*. This beautiful plant has attractive purple blossoms with a heady aroma that is hard for me and the bees to resist plunging our noses into every time we pass her in the garden. She does well in a large pot that I transfer indoors before the first frost -- in temperate climates she will grow as a perennial.

Common Name(s): Holy Basil, Tulsi, Sacred Basil, Garden Balsam, Green Tulsi, Tulasi
Botanical Name(s): *Ocimum basilicum, Ociumum tenuflorum*

Botanical Family: Lamiaceae – Mint Family
Plant Parts Used: Leaves and flowering tops
Odor Profile: Green, spicy, warming. Tulsi smells a bit like lemon, mint, licorice, and cloves all together
Flavor: Spicy, peppery, clove-like flavor
Safety Considerations: It may be prudent to restrict usage of hydrosols distilled from botanicals known for their high eugenol and estragole content during pregnancy, breastfeeding, in pediatrics, and those with ulcers or clotting disorders, until further research can be done to assess risk
Biophysical Actions: analgesic, antimicrobial, anxiolytic, carminative, expectorant, immunomodulatory, nervine

Tulsi is one of my favorite hydrosols to go into cold and flu season with. It not only supports the immune system and calms the nervous system, it also works really well in a nasal rinse and nebulizer treatment to prevent and treat upper respiratory tract infections. I've been using it a bit for my non-asthmatic clients experiencing environmental allergies and we're seeing some promising results as well.

Rose-Tulsi Cordial

We get spring, summer, and fall rose crops here in Central Texas and I count myself quite blessed with the abundance of one of my favorite aromatic flowers. Choose an unsprayed rose bush with a couple years of growth under its belt. Pick the roses at their peak — shortly after they've opened to the world and when their aroma is most strong. I find early mornings to be an ideal time to maximize flavor and aroma.

1 pint jar loosely packed rose petals
brandy
1/2 cup raw, local honey
2 ounces holy basil hydrosol

Loosely pack a pint-sized mason jar with freshly picked rose petals, pour honey over the petals and fill to the shoulders of the jar with the brandy. Seal and shake once a day for 4-6 weeks. Strain the petals and top off with the holy basil (tulsi) hydrosol. Take by the dropperful in a glass of water or use as cocktail syrup, adding it to sparkling water or prosecco.

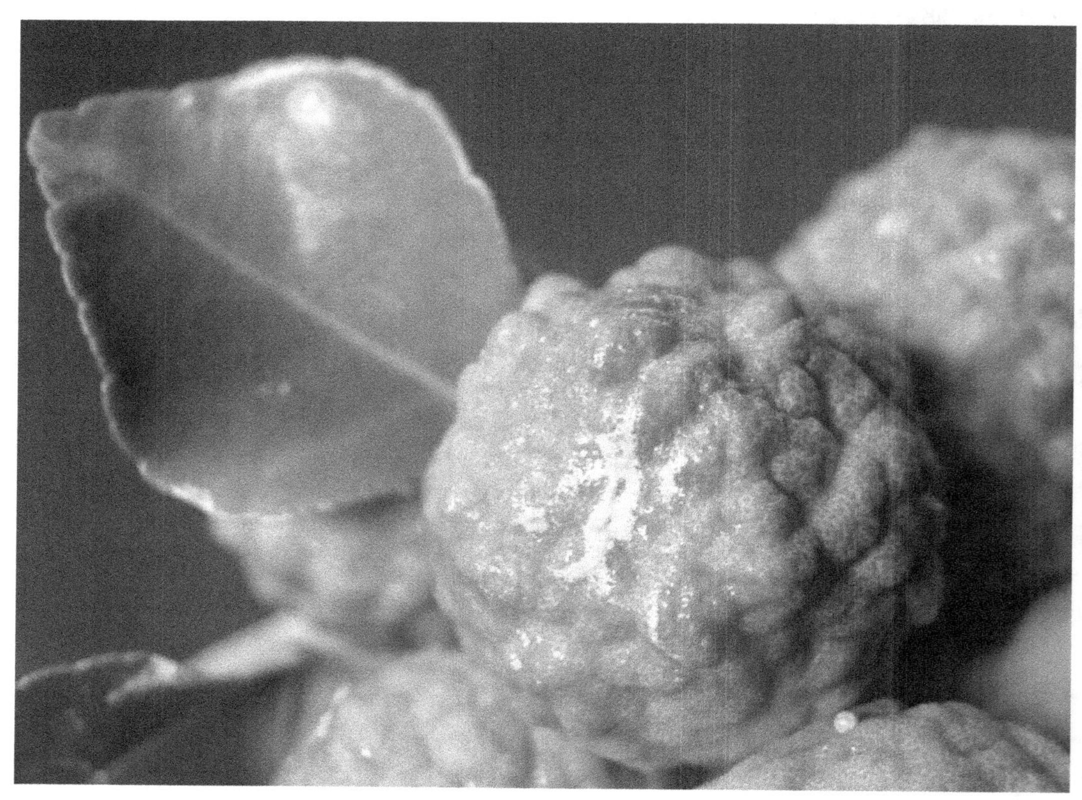

10 BERGAMOT

Bergamot is a hybrid of bitter orange (*Citrus aurantium L.*) and lime (*Citrus aurantifolia*), producing a rather inedible fruit, whose peel has been revered by Earl Grey tea drinkers since the 1800s. This citrus has a sweet, uplifting aroma to it, which is enjoyable in a glass of sparkling water or spritzed directly on the skin.

Research indicates Bergamot essential oil has an immunostimulant action (Cosentino, Luini, et al 2014), and has been classically recommended as an antidepressant (Sheppard-Hanger 1995). Jane Buckle, PhD, in her book *Clinical Aromatherapy, 3rd edition*, references a cystic fibrosis study (Borgatti et al 2011), in which the essential oil of Bergamot reduced some of the chemokines and cytokines associated with the inflammatory response in the lungs of CF patients.

Common Name(s): Bergamot
Botanical Name(s): *Citrus bergamia, Citrus aurantium ssp bergamia, Oleum bergamottae*
Botanical Family: Rutaceae (citrus family)
Plant Parts Used: Outer peel, whole fruit
Odor Profile: Floral citrusy
Flavor: Mild citrus flavor mellowed by esters
Safety Considerations: Because it is steam-distilled, the hydrosol doesn't contain furanocoumarins and therefore does not pose phototoxicity concerns
Biophysical Actions: analgesic, antibacterial, antifungal, antiviral, antitumoral, stomachic, immunostimulant, neuroprotective

Bergamot has an affinity for dispersing stagnation in the body. This makes it useful in digestive wellness plans for flatulence, loss of appetite, colic, and dyspepsia. Its immunostimulant, antibacterial, antiviral, and antifungal properties make it a useful hydrosol for sore throats, tonsillitis, and other infections of the oral cavity. Consider pairing it with Fragonia™ to soothe a sore, scratchy throat.

Seattle Fog Latte

My friends in Seattle live on Queen Anne hill and when we visited them in the autumn, they took us to Kerry Park, with a breathtaking view of the city skyline, as fog rolled in off Puget Sound. I was inspired to make this beverage after that trip with some loose leaf black tea we found in Pike Place. I think of rainy days with a good book and cat snuggles with the recipe. I use Bergamot hydrosol regularly for cases of seasonal affective disorder (SAD) during the long, grey days of winter. You can make a reasonable facsimile of this recipe with rooibos (I add a few drops of cinnamon hydrosol too).

1 black tea bag
4 ounces hot water
4 ounces whole milk
1/2 teaspoon Bergamot hydrosol
honey, to taste

Steep the tea bag in the hot water. In the meanwhile, warm the milk in the microwave or on the stovetop until hot. Froth the milk using a small French press or a handheld frother until foamy. Remove the tea bag and stir in honey and bergamot hydrosol; add milk foam. Serve.

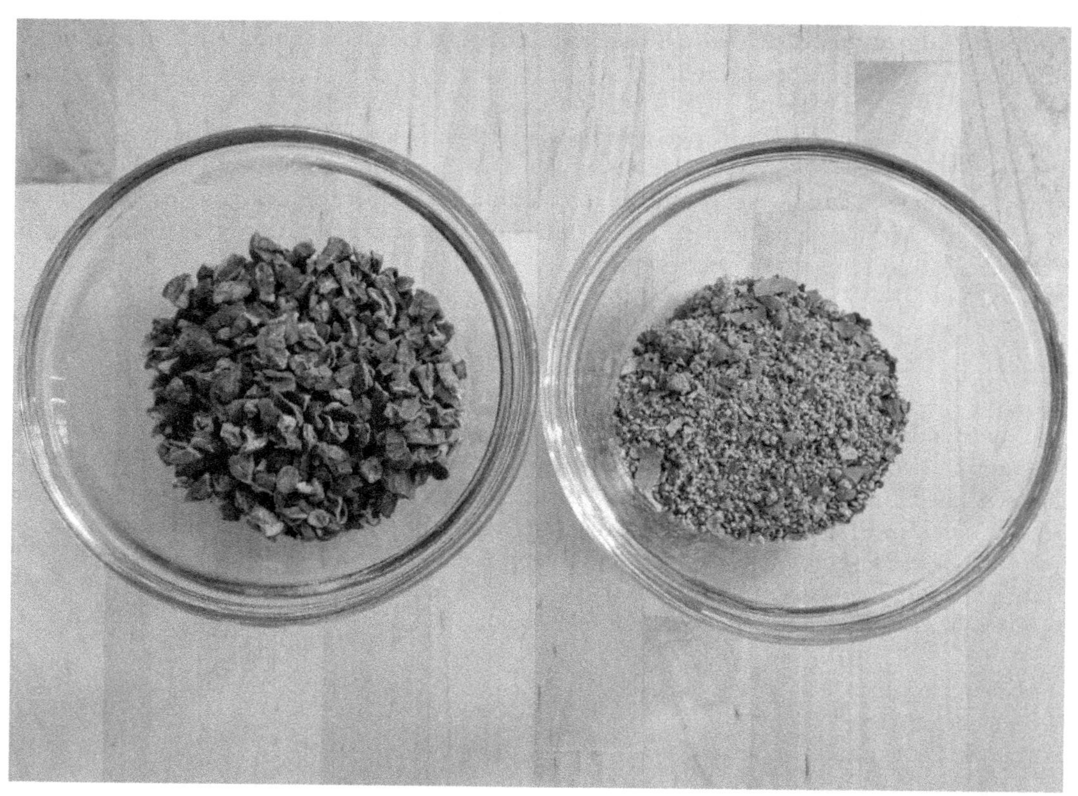

11 CACAO

Cacao is an evergreen tree that grows up with 4-8 meters (13-26 feet) tall in the tropical regions of South America up through Mexico. The seeds, known as a cocoa beans, are used to make chocolate and cocoa powder.

Common Name(s): Cacao, Cocoa
Botanical Name(s): *Theobroma cacao*
Botanical Family: Malvaceae (mallow family)
Plant Parts Used: Seeds (cocoa bean)
Odor Profile: Chocolatey
Flavor: Earthy ganache
Safety Considerations: None known
Biophysical Actions: antioxidant, cognitive stimulant

The hydrosol has a lovely chocolatey aroma that I've found quite useful for curbing cravings during sugar fasts or in cases where sugar intake needs to be restricted due to diabetes. Try adding a teaspoon to a mug of warm water to enjoy as a hot cocoa alternative, or pair it with an espresso and steamed non-dairy milk for a low calorie "mocha."

My personal favorite application though is as a face toner, there's just something that tickles me about spraying chocolate water on my face in the morning to set the mood for a really good day.

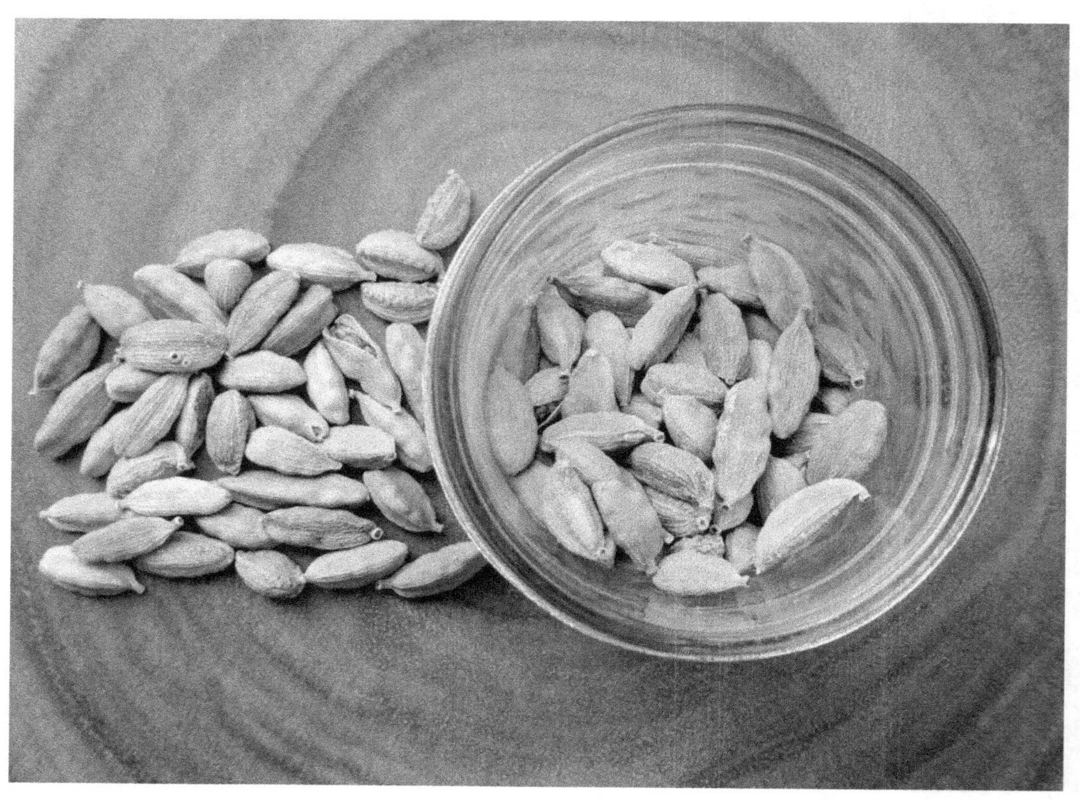

12 CARDAMOM

Cardamom is an aromatic perennial native to Southern India. The plant grows 2-4 meters (6-13 feet) in height, producing long linear lanceolate, or straight-narrow leaves. Spikes produce white to pale violet flowers and the fruit pods are green, with three sides containing several black and dark brown seeds.

Common Name(s): Cardamom, Cardamum
Botanical Name(s): *Elettaria cardamomum*
Botanical Family: Zingiberaceae (ginger family)
Plant Parts Used: Seeds
Odor Profile: Spicy, warm, sweet, with floral and camphoraceous undertones
Flavor: Spicy, earthy, citrusy
Safety Considerations: None known
Biophysical Actions: cephalic, stimulant, warming

The hydrosol of cardamom is warming and spicy, which works well for cold, damp, and weak conditions. I use it for cases of sluggishness or stagnation in the digestive and circulatory systems, from flatulence and loss of appetite to poor circulation resulting in weak muscle tone and cold hands and feet year-round. The hydrosol has been well accepted by my clients with anorexia nervosa and seems to both stimulate appetite as well as ease lethargy and the cognitive deficiency that makes concentration and memory recall a challenge for this condition. It is also one of my go-to remedies for my senior clients, who are struggling with depression or listlessness and wear sweaters in August. I use cardamom hydrosol in my wild cherry cough syrup to help loosen stagnant mucus in the lower respiratory tract.

I have Scandinavian ancestors and use this as an excuse to explain away my obsession for all things cardamom. Try spritzing fresh, chopped mango pieces with the hydrosols or add a few drops to your coffee. This cardamom syrup recipe below can be used to drizzle over desserts, fresh fruit, or in your favorite cocktails and mocktails.

Cardamom Syrup

If you want an even stronger cardamom flavor, you can simmer 3 cardamom pods in the sugar syrup phase. I often triple this batch so I have enough on hand for a couple of weeks' worth of recipes.

1/3 cup water
1/3 cup sugar
2 teaspoons (10 mls) cardamom

In a small saucepan, bring the sugar and water to a simmer on medium high. Reduce heat to low and stir for 3 minutes. Cool. Whisk in 10 mls cardamom hydrosol. Use the syrup to pour over roasted plums, peaches, or nectarines before serving. Also makes a great tea or cocktail syrup: add an ounce to an old-fashioned, or half an ounce to a glass of nettle tea.

Spiced Wine

Mulled, or spiced wine is a lovely winter treat after an afternoon of snowshoeing, skiing, or ice skating. It is commonly served around Christmas and Solstice. I enjoy a bit of spiced wine whenever the weather and my mood calls for it.

1 bottle red wine
5 cups apple cider
1/3 cup honey
2 sticks of cinnamon (or 5 mls of cinnamon hydrosol)
1 orange, zested and juiced
5 whole cloves
3 star anise
5 mls (1 teaspoon) cardamom hydrosol

In a medium sized pot, add wine, juice, and spices. Bring to a boil and immediately reduce heat to simmer for 15-30 minutes. Remove from heat and add honey and hydrosol(s). Serve warm.

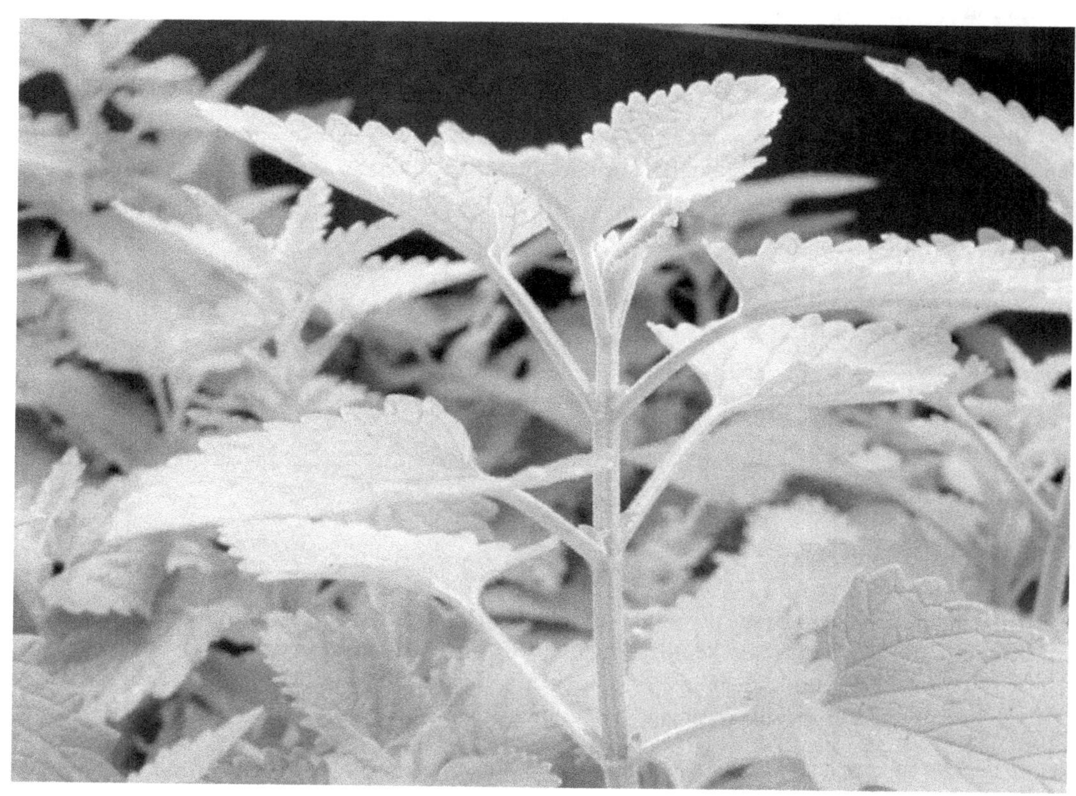

13 CATNIP

Catnip is an herbal perennial with the square stems and terminal flower spikes we see in other members of the mint family. It grows well in many climates, and is native to the dry and temperate climes of the Mediterranean region.

The hydrosol has a pleasant, minty-lemony-herbaceous aroma and flavor that is pleasurable to both felines and humans.

Common Name(s): Catnip, Catmint
Botanical Name(s): *Nepeta cataria*
Botanical Family: Lamiaceae (mint family)
Plant Parts Used: Aerial parts
Odor Profile: Mint-lemoney
Flavor: Initially cool, minty, with a faint lemon taste, warms with additional sips

Safety Considerations: Avoid in first trimester of pregnancy, due to slight uterine stimulant action

Biophysical Actions: calmative, digestive stimulant, emmenagogue, insect repellent, relaxant

Catnip hydrosol is calming and relaxing for both adults and children, making it a good choice for bedtime wellness plans to slow down the mental chatter and ease into sleep. I recommend parents traveling through different time zones with children pack some catnip to either add to a pre-bedtime glass of water or to spritz the pillow cases at the hotel or guest room to encourage easier transitions for the immature circadian rhythm. It's also useful for unsettled tummies, which makes it a handy first-aid remedy when traveling or at home.

As a gentle emmenagogue, catnip hydrosol is useful for irregular menstrual cycles. I recommend clients start taking 5 mls of the hydrosol in a glass of water before bedtime a few days before the new moon for 5-6 nights and using nightlight stimulation around the full moon to stimulate ovulation. Barrier method contraception is appropriate during cycle regulation attempts to avoid an unplanned pregnancy.

The hydrosol makes for a very gentle mosquito repellent for young children. I recommend diluting it with an equal amount of water, adding to a bottle with a spray nozzle, and spraying the stroller blanket or carseat upholstery for children under 12 months of age.

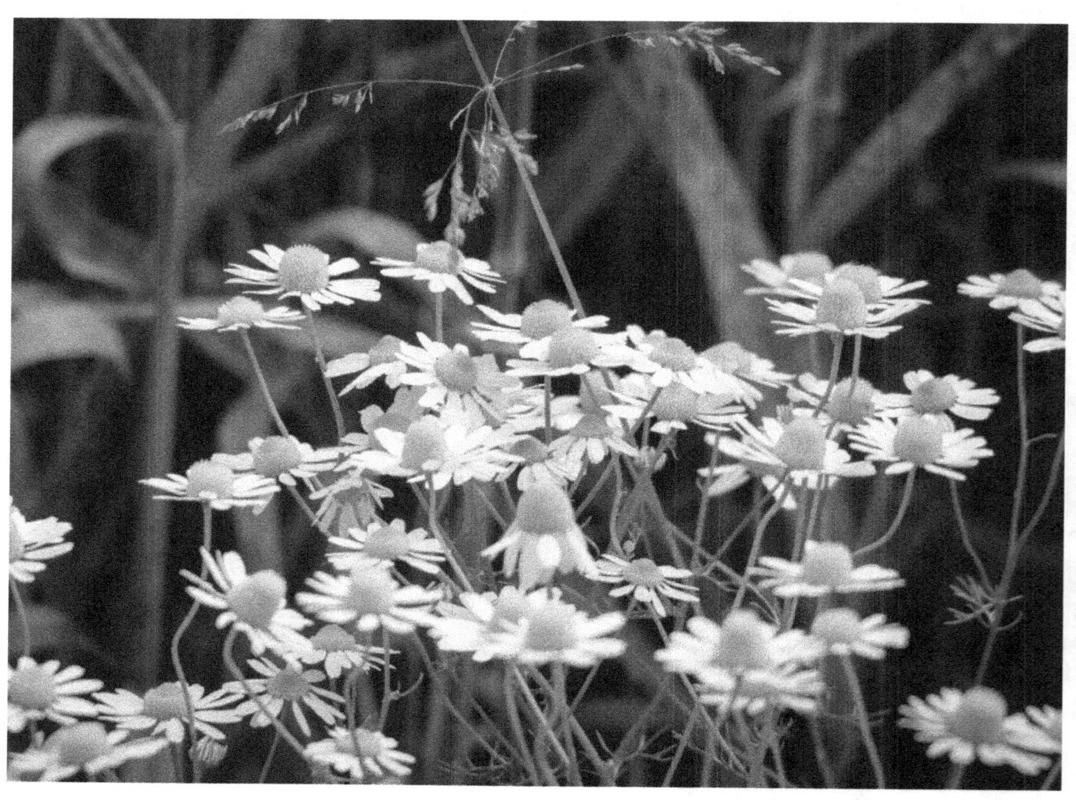

14 CHAMOMILE, GERMAN

German Chamomile is a perennial herb with hairless, branching stems that grow up to half a meter (2 feet) in height, bearing small white flowers resembling the daisy.

While Germany doesn't grow this chamomile commercially anymore, it has been naturalized in other areas of Europe, Australia, and the United States.

Common Name(s): German Chamomile, Blue Chamomile, Wild Chamomile, Hungarian Chamomile
Botanical Name(s): *Matricaria recutita, Chamomilla recutita, Matricria chamomilla*
Botanical Family: Asteraceae (daisy family)
Plant Parts Used: Aerial parts of flowering plant
Odor Profile: Sweet herbaceous, hint of apples
Flavor: Floral herbaceous with slight bitter end that isn't wholly unpleasant

Safety Considerations: None known
Biophysical Actions: antihistamine, anti-inflammatory, anodyne, sedative

German Chamomile is a cooling hydrosol that soothes inflamed skin and mucosal membranes. Undiluted, it can be used to calm fiery skin patterns like dermatitis, eczema, psoriasis, and rosacea. It also makes a great first aid tool for kitchen burns, sunburns, new-sandals blisters, insect bites and stings, and heat rashes. I recommend it for clients who are receiving radiation therapy for tumors and cancerous cells. It can be used one of two ways for radiation burns: 1) straight out of the refrigerator, spritzed onto the affected area, before applying a cream or oil, or 2) as the water base of an aromatic gel applied to the affected area as needed.

Hot, throbbing hemorrhoids and gluteal fold irritation get cooling relief with a 25-50% solution in a squeezable peri bottle. Use the hydrosol rinse on the affected area several times a day, especially following a bowel movement, and the let the area drip dry. A soothing hip bath can bring comfort and relief as well – fill the bathtub to hip height and pour in a cup of hydrosol, soak for 15-20 minutes and gently towel off. The 25% dilution is also lovely for diaper rash and heat rash in babies and toddlers.

Varicose and spider veins can benefit from the cooling, soothing action of German Chamomile hydrosol. Soak a cloth in the hydrosol, wring out until just damp, and cover the affected area. This is safe to use during pregnancy and I've had many clients who found this, paired with peppermint hydrosol, was what got them through the last days of pregnancy when hot, angry veins were so uncomfortable.

Aloe Chamomile Sunburn Soother

15 mls German Chamomile hydrosol
15 mls Aloe Vera gel

Mix hydrosol and gel together in a small vessel. Apply to sunburned skin with a cosmetic brush, cotton round, or gentle fingers.

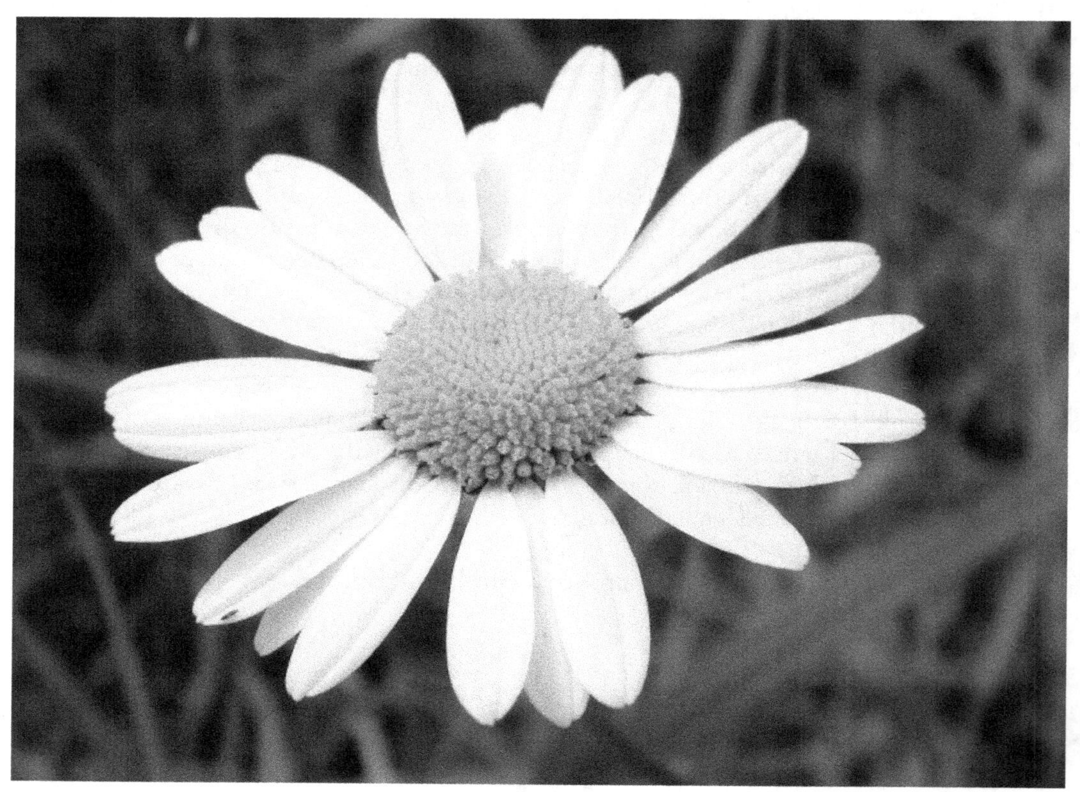

15 CHAMOMILE, ROMAN

Roman Chamomile is a much shorter plant than Matricaria (German Chamomile), but has larger daisy-like white flowers. It is one of the oldest known medicinal herbs -- dedicated to the Egyptian sun god Ra, and used as an sacred plant in ancient Egypt. During the Tudor era, this flowering herb was used as ground cover, creating floral-apple scented lawns.

The British Herbal Pharmacopeia indicates the herb's uses for nervousness, restlessness, irritability in children, anorexia, vomiting in pregnancy, and flatulent dyspepsia associated with mental distress.

Common Name(s): Roman Chamomile, English Chamomile, Lawn Chamomile
Botanical Name(s): *Anthemis nobilis, Chamaemelum nobile*

Botanical Family: Asteraceae (daisy family)
Plant Parts Used: Aerial parts of flowering plant
Odor Profile: Fruity – reminiscent of apples or pineapples
Flavor: Fruity-floral with a slight herbaceous quality
Safety Considerations: Persons with ragweed allergies may react to Roman Chamomile as well(a patch test would be prudent)
Biophysical Actions: anodyne, antispasmodic, anxiolytic, sedative

Roman Chamomile is a soothing hydrosol for the nervous and digestive systems. I turn to this chamomile for mild tension headaches or headaches stemming from a too-rich dinner. Its anxiolytic, or antianxiety, action is very calming in times of acute stress – I nearly went through a 4-ounce bottle of this hydrosol during our last move, when I felt like I'd been transported to a Lemony Snicket book: the truck rental gave us a van which spelled out a life size game of Tetris, then the movers locked the keys in the van, then we had to bring in two more vehicles to meet the deadline... Needless to say a bath with a couple of ounces of the hydrosol and 10 mls (2 teaspoons) in my bedtime glass of water was the only thing to bring my nerves out of the rafters.

Clients with generalized anxiety disorders and insomnia have had good success adding Roman Chamomile and Neroli hydrosol to their wellness plans to assist with troubled sleep and panic attacks. It has made a huge difference for a couple of clients to take a bottle of water with these hydrosols added to it to their talk therapy appointments with their mental health professionals when challenging subjects are addressed.

It is also a useful hydrosol for inflammation of the eyelid (Valnet, J 1980). Just soak a cotton round in the hydrosol and lie it across the affected eyelid while lying down. My postpartum clients have found this hydrosol helpful for treating dry, cracked, and sore nipples, by spritzing the areola and nipple with the hydrosol and then following with a cream or oil.

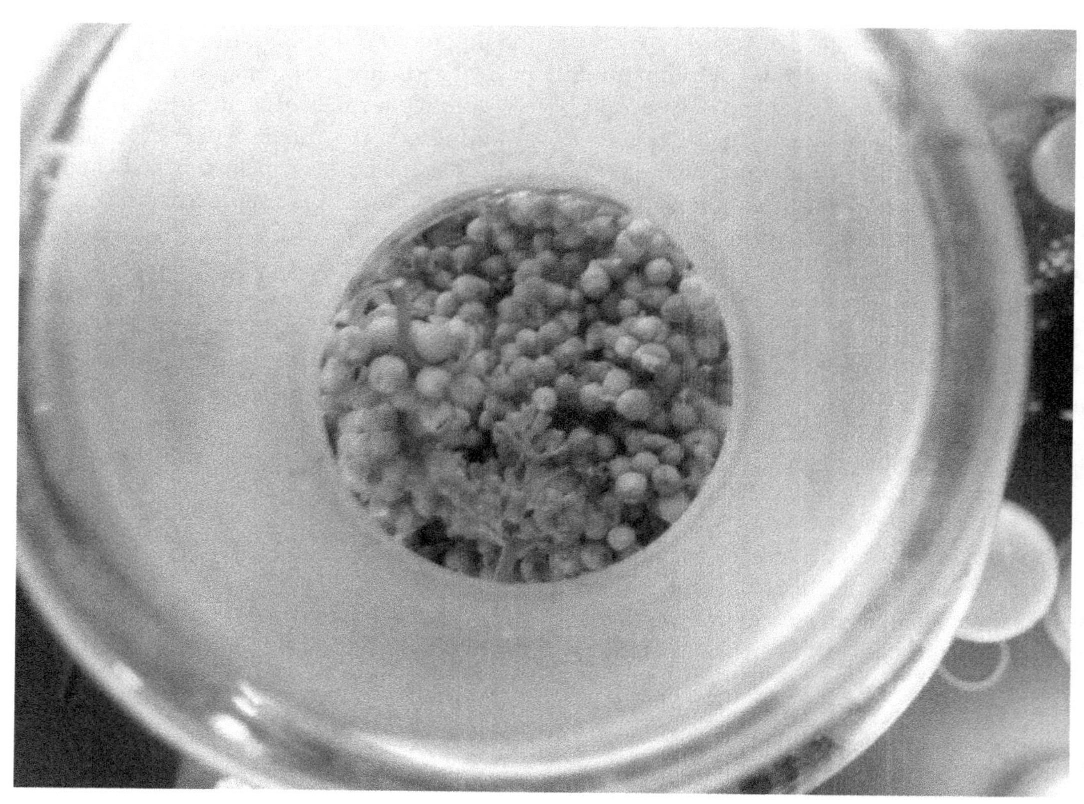

16 CHASTE TREE (VITEX)

A small tree with lance shaped leaves and purple flowers, native to the Mediterranean, but cultivated in temperate climates around the globe. Dioscorides recommended Vitex berries to lower libido (Schulz et al., 1998) and Pliny wrote that soldiers' wives whose beds were strewn with the berries had been faithful to their husbands away at battle (Hobbs, 1996). There is no scientific evidence that Vitex has an anaphrodesiac or libido-reducing action to it.

The herb has a historical use for treating constipation, fevers, flatulence, and hangovers.

Common Name(s): Chaste Tree, Vitex, Chasteberry, Lilac Chastetree, Monk's Berry
Botanical Name(s): *Vitex agnus castus*
Botanical Family: Verbenaceae (verbena family)

Plant Parts Used: leaves or berries
Odor Profile: Pungent with a bitter-herbaceous quality
Flavor: Strongly bitter
Safety Considerations: Interacts with hormonal contraceptives, likely unpleasant for men, avoid in pregnancy and children
Biophysical Actions: hormone regulator

I use vitex hydrosol primarily to ease hot flashes, night sweats, and relieve mild mood swings in menopausal clients. We've done some early experiments with clients to see if there's much benefit to adding the hydrosol to fertility clients with luteal phase defect, but I haven't had enough cases to show results. It does appear to be a gentle support tool for those with poly cystic ovary syndrome (PCOS).

Night Sweat Linen Spray

My menopausal clients love this simple linen spray! They keep the bottle stored in the fridge until they're ready to use it then spritz down their bed sheets where their torso will be, as that is where they produce the most heat.

30 mls Vitex hydrosol
30 mls Lavender or Marjoram hydrosol

Pour hydrosols into a 2-ounce bottle, shake to combine. Spritz linens; then return to fridge.

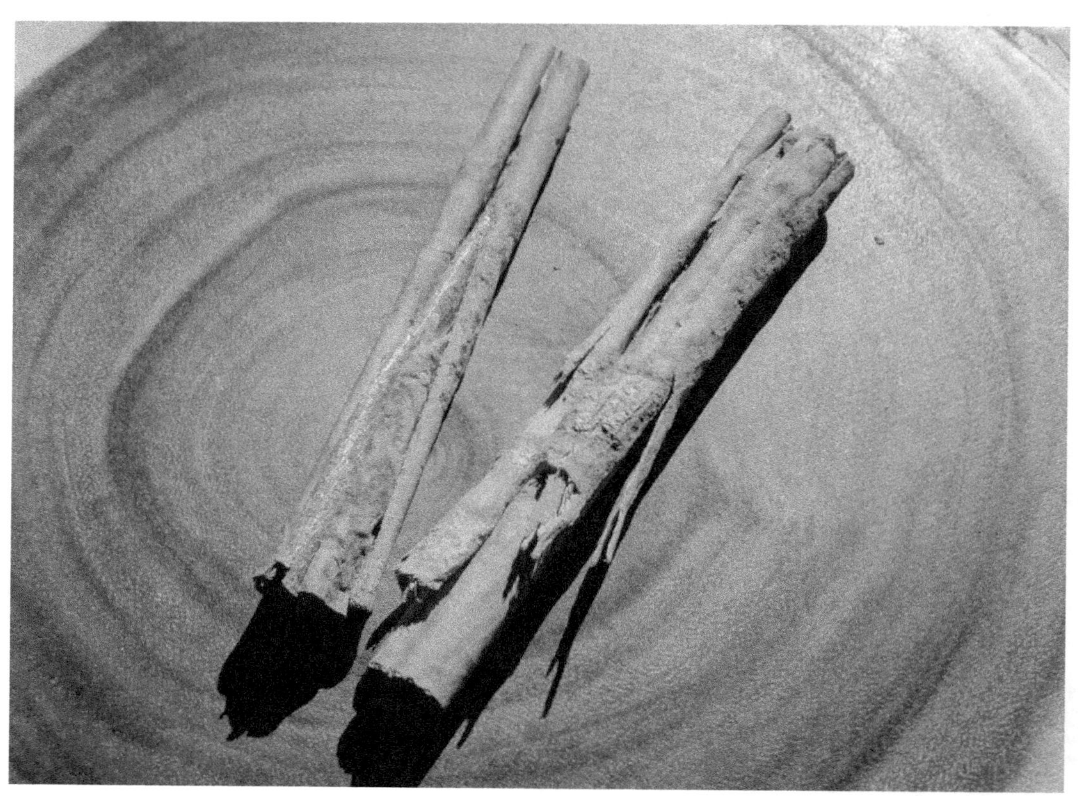

17 CINNAMON BARK

Cinnamon is an evergreen tree in the laurel family, native to Sri Lanka and now cultivated in Seychelles and Madagascar. The tree reaches 10-15 meters (30-50 feet) in height, with ovate-oblong leaves and green colored flowers. The bark is harvested from the young shoots.

Cinnamon essential oil is a high skin sensitizer and I've yet to find a use for the hydrosol in its undiluted form.

Common Name(s): Cinnamon, Ceylon Cinnamon
Botanical Name(s): *Cinnamomum verum, Cinnamomum zeylanicum*
Botanical Family: Lauraceae (laurel family)
Plant Parts Used: Bark
Odor Profile: Pungent, sweet-spicy
Flavor: Very pungent, sweet, peppery

Safety Considerations: Irritant, skin sensitizer, the essential oil is contraindicated for pregnancy, children, breastfeeding, and cautioned for those on anticoagulants, diabetic medications, following major surgery, bleeding disorders, and peptic ulcers
Biophysical Actions: analgesic, antiseptic, antimicrobial, rubefacient

Cinnamon bark hydrosol has a pleasant, pungent aroma and is just the thing when you need a strongly warming hydrosol for cold, aching joints and muscles. Add 5-10 mls to a foot soak for cold feet that have been standing outdoors in freezing temps shoveling snow or watching a football game in the freezing rain.

The hydrosol makes a nice mouth rinse for gums with poor circulation (pale, receding), or a gargle at the first sign of a throat infection.

Horchata

Growing up, I spent time in Central Mexico with my grandparents on Lake Chapala. Horchata was one of my favorite beverages to order at the corner market in the village and in Guadalajara. I don't like the grittiness of horchatas that have had ground cinnamon added, since it cakes up the bottom of the glass like brown sand. 5-10 mls of hydrosol have been just the thing to give a rich cinnamon flavor and aroma without the sludge of the powdered spice or the weak flavor from adding a stick or two to the water.

1 cup white rice, rinsed
8 cups water, divided
½ cup sugar, to taste
Cinnamon hydrosol, to taste

Combine the rice with 4 cups of the water in the blender. Pulse or blend until rice has broken into a coarse meal. Transfer to a pitcher adding the other 4 cups of water and let sit at room temperature for a minimum of 3 hours. Strain through a fine mesh sieve, a nut milk or jelly bag, or layers of cheesecloth. Make a simple syrup of a bit of the rice milk and the sugar, cool and combine. Add cinnamon hydrosol. Chill to serve.

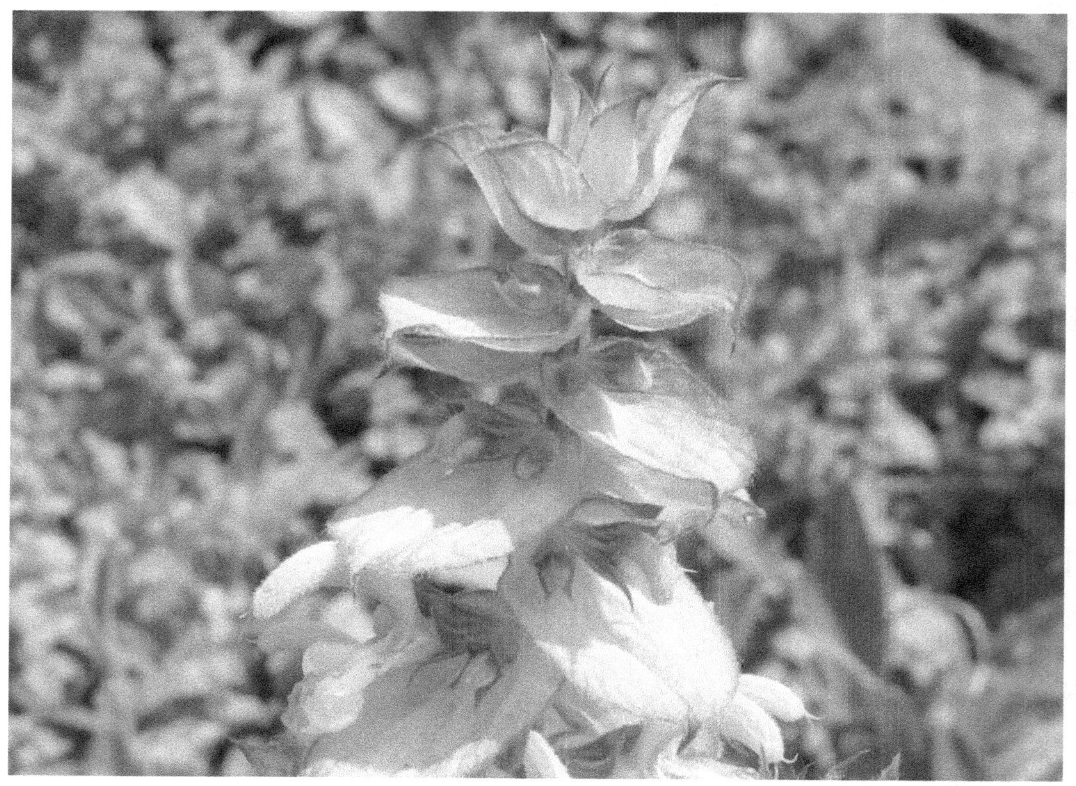

18 CLARY SAGE

Clary Sage is an erect biennial herb native to the Mediterranean region and southern Europe. It grows up to a meter (3-4 feet) in height, with broad-ovate, green leaves and lilac to blue colored flowers. The plant received its name, *Sclarea*, which means clear or bright, from the traditional use for clearing foreign bodies from the eye. Culpepper wrote of using the herbal form of the seed to draw 'motes' from the eye, as well as to draw out splinters and thorns embedded in the skin. Used as an alternative to beer, Grieve claims it gave an almost insane exhilaration, swiftly followed by a severe headache. Clary Sage is grown for its essential oil, absolute, and hydrosol. The absolute is used to produce a synthetic ambergris-like compound for the perfume industry.

Common Name(s): Clary Sage, Muscatel Sage
Botanical Name(s): *Salvia sclarea*
Botanical Family: Lamiaceae (mint family)

Plant Parts Used: Leaves and flowering tops
Odor Profile: Sweet-herbaceous, slightly woody and balsamic
Flavor: Herbaceous, earthy, woody
Safety Considerations: None known
Biophysical Actions: antispasmodic, nervous restorative, relaxant

Clary Sage hydrosol has a nice range of uses from skin care to wellness to culinary. I've used it in the nebulizer, paired with cypress for asthma and coughing fits, where the diaphragm is overly taxed and the client is exhausted from trying to catch their breath. The essential oil is favored for women's health and, while neither the oil nor the hydrosol have mechanisms to bring on labor, I do like offering the hydrosol as a tonic for my postdates pregnant clients to relax and prepare for baby's signal.

My intuitive friends use Clary Sage hydrosol to tap into the third eye chakra to enhance visions and inner meditative work. I've found a spritz over the face before a meditation session to be comforting, supportive, and have come out of meditation with a giggle bubbling up from diaphragm.

In the kitchen, this hydrosol can be used to flavor cold soups or in sweet vinaigrettes for a fruit salad.

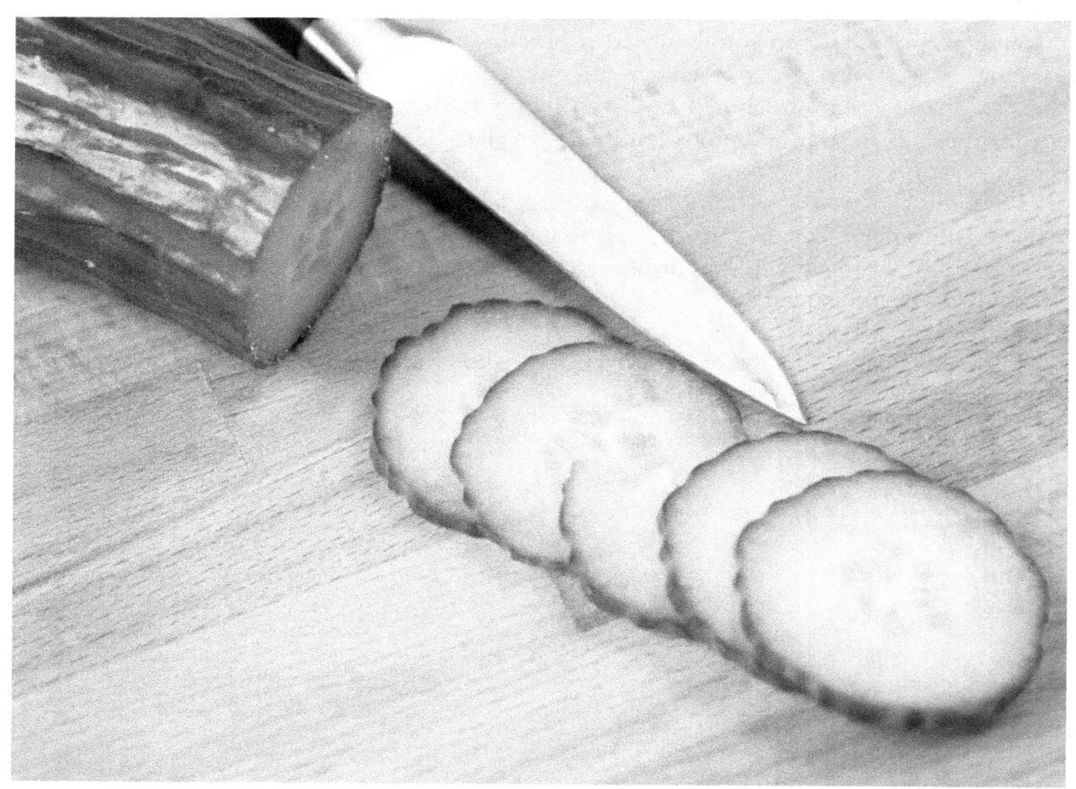

19 CUCUMBER

Cucumber is a creeping vine you've probably grown in your own backyard garden at some point. Raw cucumber is over 90% water and lends itself nicely to a true hydrosol distillation.

Common Name(s): Cucumber
Botanical Name(s): *Cucumis sativus*
Botanical Family: Curcurbitaceae (gourd family)
Plant Parts Used: Fruit (vegetable)
Odor Profile: Mild, green vegetal aroma
Flavor: Tastes like a milder version of the vegetable, sweet and mild
Safety Considerations: None known
Biophysical Actions: cooling, hydrating

Cucumber hydrosol has a fresh, green scent that smells just like the vegetable. It is cooling and hydrating, making it a great choice for hot, tired eyes in an eye compress, as well as for everyday skincare during warm months. Try adding a bit to a glass of water after gardening with a few crushed, seasonal berries. Delish!

Hydrosol Eye Compress

Soak two cotton rounds in a teaspoon each of chilled cucumber, lavender, or rose hydrosol. Place over closed eyes and enjoy the cooling comfort. Consider this application after eye strain at the computer or mobile electronic device, during allergy season when eyes are itchy and puffy, or just when you need a little TLC for your peepers.

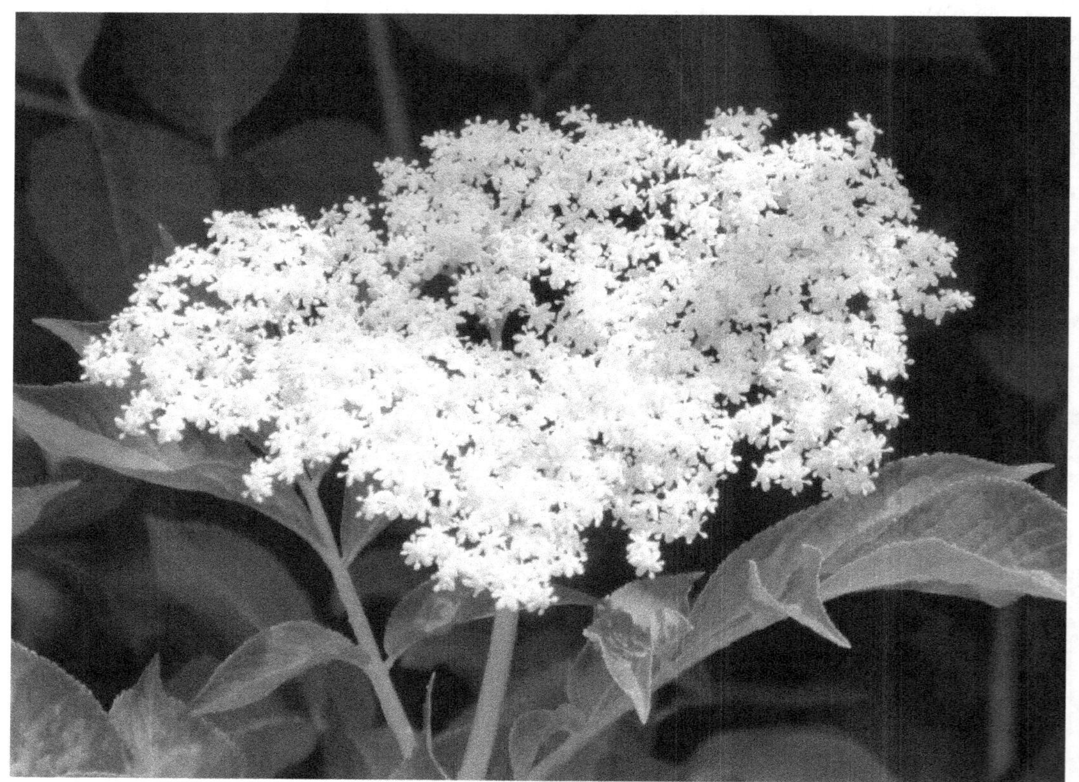

20 ELDERFLOWER

Elder is a deciduous shrub or small tree growing up to 6 meters (20 feet) in height. Perhaps best known for its glossy dark purple berries used to prevent and treat influenza virus, the flowers make a delicious cordial and wine. St-Germain is a mildly alcoholic sparkling elderflower liqueur available on the commercial market in the United States.

Elderflower as an herbal tea is used for feverish colds to produce a sweat and ease catarrh congestion in the airways (Bradley 1992).

Common Name(s): Elder, Elderberry
Botanical Name(s): *Sambucus nigra and Sambucus cerulea*
Botanical Family: (moschatel family)
Plant Parts Used: Fruit (vegetable)
Odor Profile: Mild, sweet floral

Flavor: Sweet floral with a hint of green
Safety Considerations: None known
Biophysical Actions: anti-inflammatory, antiviral, diaphoretic, diuretic

Nigra is more common in Europe, while Cerulea is more common in North America, but both are used interchangeably for their medicinal effects. Elderflower hydrosol is one of those lightly floral hydrosols that will have you falling in love with aromatic waters!

Elderflower hydrosol is a very gentle antiviral. I enjoy it in a glass of water leading up to cold and flu season. It's also a mild diuretic and will gently act on the waters of the body.

Recovery Popsicles

Therapeutic popsicles can be comfort food after a night of vomiting, teething, or influenza. I like using elderflower hydrosol during or following the common cold, especially in children. Avoid Elderflower hydrosol in cases of vomiting, as the diuretic properties don't support a body experiencing dehydration. Be sure to look for a fruit juice with no added sugars.

2 cups peach juice
10 mls elderflower hydrosol

Combine juice and hydrosol in a large measuring cup. Using the cup's spout, pour mixture into popsicle molds. Freeze until solid, about six hours.

For other recovery popsicle ideas, consider:
- Teething – Chamomile hydrosol and white grape or apple juice
- Post stomach flu – Ginger hydrosol and pear or peach juice
- Post hangover – Peppermint hydrosol and white grape or apple juice

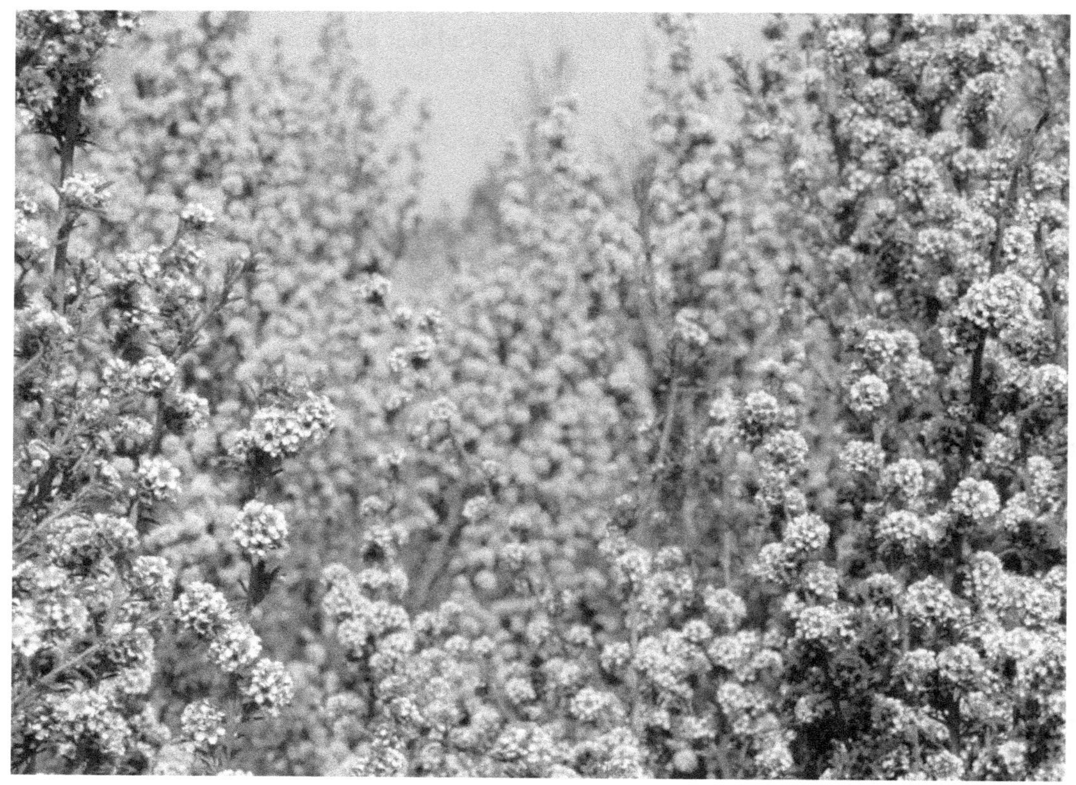

21 FRAGONIA™

Fragonia is a flowering shrub native to Australia that reaches 2.4 meters (7.9 feet) in height and has aromatic, white blossoms.

There is one primary farm that is making Fragonia commercially-available and they do not distill for a true hydrosol. However, it is an above-average biowaste and does produce a very nice hydrosol. I would love to see an authentic hydrosol of Fragonia on the market in the very near future, as it is a beautiful product with a lot of promise for many different types of wellness plans.

Common Name(s): Fragonia
Botanical Name(s): *Agonis fragrans*
Botanical Family: Myrtaceae (myrtle family)
Plant Parts Used: Flowering tops with leaves and twigs

Odor Profile: Floral-phenolic
Flavor: Pungent on the front end, but softens to a nice phenolic floral
Safety Considerations: None known
Biophysical Actions: analgesic, antimicrobial

Fragonia is on my go-to list for jet lag, sore throats, arthritis, back pain, autoimmune conditions with infectious components, and respiratory tract infections from sinusitis to bronchitis. I use it in nebulizers for jet lag and respiratory infections, in the bath for back pain and aching joints, in water for my clients with Crohn's and Lyme's disease, and in a honey syrup for throat and oral cavity infections.

Aromatic Honey Syrup

This honey syrup is great for soothing a sore throat during times of seasonal illness. In cold climates, the honey may need to be gently warmed – put the glass jar of honey in a saucepan of warm water and let it sit for 30 minutes or so until it is pourable again.

30 mls raw, local honey
15 mls Fragonia™ hydrosol
5 mls Bergamot hydrosol

Bring hydrosol to room temperature and whisk it into the liquid honey. Refrigerate for a couple of hours. Add a teaspoon or more of the syrup to a glass of warm water.

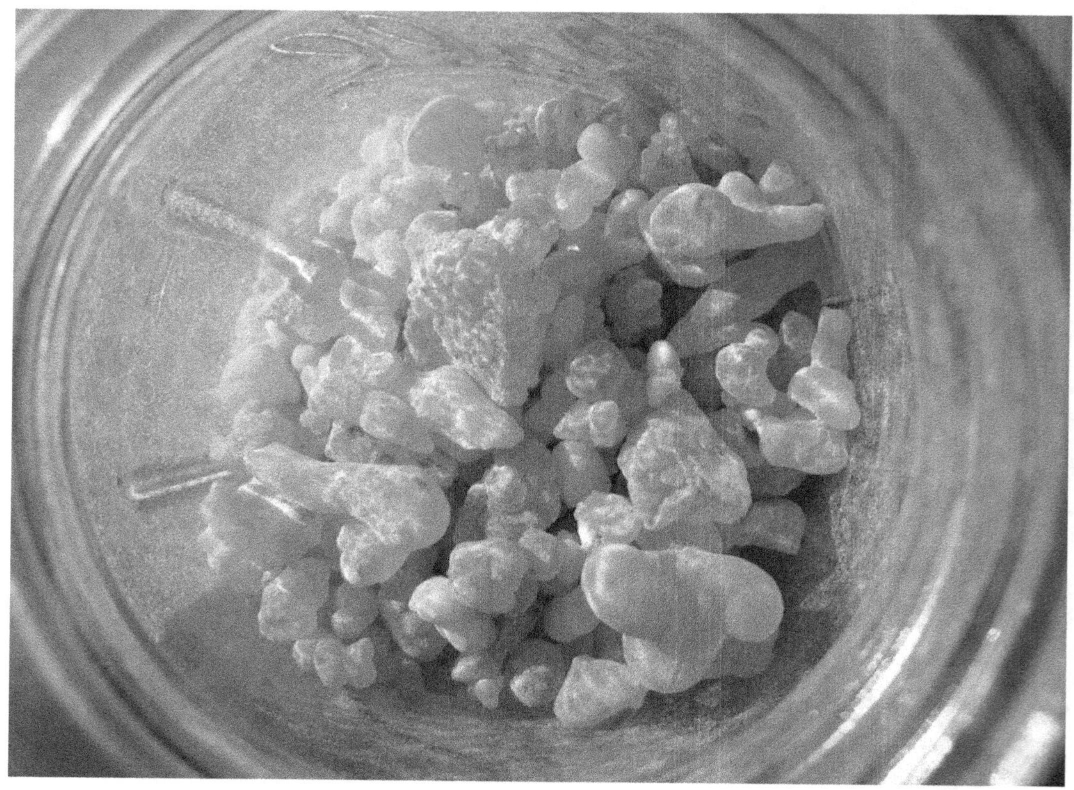

22 FRANKINCENSE

Boswellia carterii is a small, evergreen tree that grows up to 6 meters (20 feet) in height, with papery, peeling bark and creamy-white to pale pink, five-petaled flowers that appear in the spring. Incisions are made into the bark of the tree, which then exudes a milky white sap, slowly congealing into yellowish teardrops that can be harvested directly from the tree or off the ground where they've fallen. The hydrosol is distilled from resin, though the biowaste from essential oil distillation is often sold as a hydrosol.

Frankincense has been used in religious festivals and ceremonies since antiquity. Historically, the herbal extract has been used as a cough medicine for asthma. In China, it was used in the treatment of leprosy. Traditional medicine systems, including Siddha, Unani, and Ayurveda, use the resin as plant medicine.

Common Name(s): Frankincense, Olibanum, Luban

Botanical Name(s): *Boswellia carterii, Boswellia sacra*
Botanical Family: Burseraceae (incense tree or torchwood family)
Plant Parts Used: Resin
Odor Profile: Woody terpenic resinous
Flavor: Woody medicinal balsamic
Safety Considerations: None known
Biophysical Actions: analgesic, antimicrobial

Frankincense hydrosol is commonly used for meditative and spiritual practices and ceremonies. Spritz a room to energetically clear it or prepare for prayer, yoga, or meditation. It's also indicated for skin formulations — one client spritzed her hands daily for a few months to fade the brown pigmentation spots from decades of sun exposure.

Frankincense Gel Serum

This serum can be used on the hands and face to combat environmental damage to the skin, while also hydrating in the summer and winter.

60 mls Frankincense hydrosol
650 mg Xanthan or Sclerotium gum
600 mg glucanolactone and sodium benzoate

In a medium-sized bowl, gently heat the hydrosol until it is lukewarm. Add the powdered gum and the GSB preservative and whisk until smooth. Use a cosmetic brush, cotton pad, or sponge to apply a thin coat to the face, paying extra attention to areas that need more hydration.

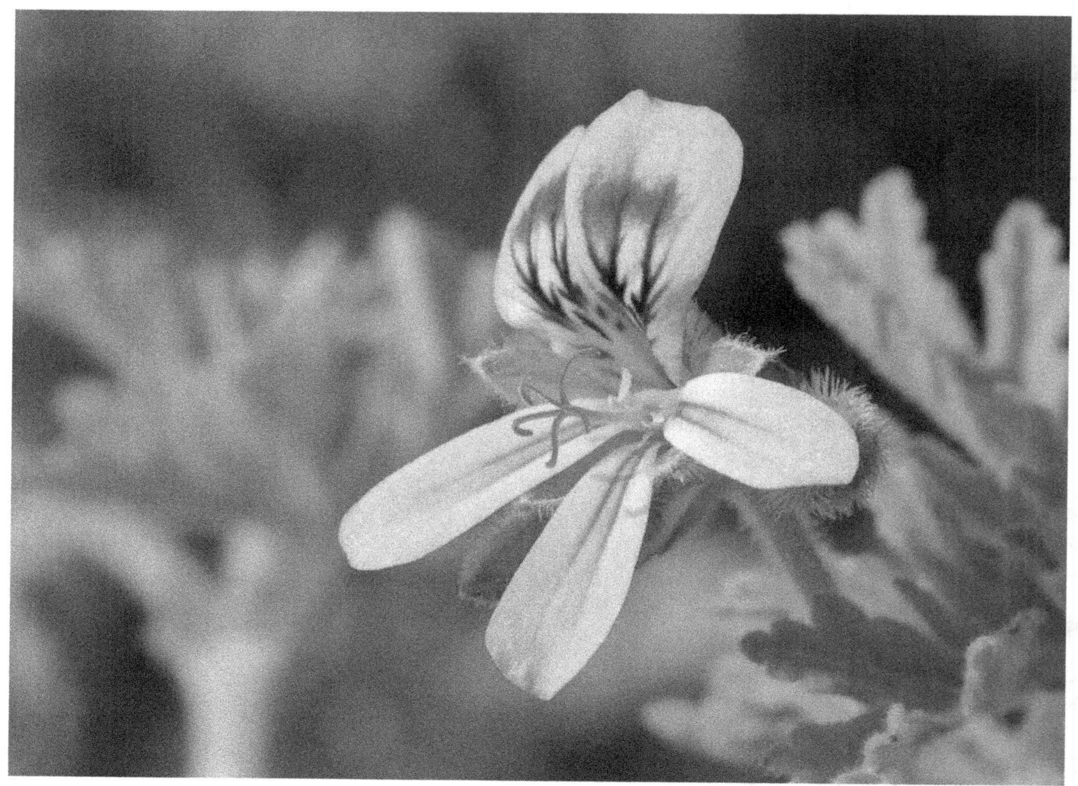

23 GERANIUM

Geranium is an aromatic, perennial shrub that reaches 1 meter (2-3 feet) in height, with serrated leaves and small pink flowers. The aroma is floral, rosy-sweet, with a green-fruity hint, thanks to its diverse ester constituents. You'll find the hydrosol isn't as fragrant as the essential oil, but does itself justice in the fragrance department nonetheless.

Valnet mentions that Geranium was used by the ancients to treat wounds, bone fractures, and cancers. French chemist Recluz is credited as the first person to distill the leaves of geranium in 1819. Popular for women's reproductive and hormonal health support, geranium has been used for premenstrual syndrome, menopausal hot flashes, estrogen-progesterone deficiencies, and menstrual cycle imbalances.

Common Name(s): Geranium, Rose Geranium, Rose-Scented Geranium
Botanical Name(s): *Pelargonium graveolens, Pelargonium odoratissimum, Pelargonium x asperum*

Botanical Family: Geraniaceae (geranium or cranesbill family)
Plant Parts Used: Leaves, flowers, stalks
Odor Profile: Rosey floral
Flavor: Sweet floral with hint of citrus and green-herbaceous
Safety Considerations: The essential oil is cautioned in interacting with diabetes medication. It is poorly tolerated in persons with high sensitivity to floral odorants (those with multiple chemical sensitivities for example)
Biophysical Actions: antidepressant, anxiolytic, mental stimulant

Geranium hydrosol brings cooling relief to clients with hot flashes and night sweats, it pairs well with Chaste Tree hydrosol, as a body mist in a spritz bottle. In the bath, it eases the aches and discomforts of the lower pelvis before a menstrual period and in a glass of water eases premenstrual feelings of anxiousness and depression. I like to pair it with Cacao hydrosol for food cravings in adolescent and adult female clients who enjoy the floral chocolate flavor. It makes a delicious addition to sparkling water with or without added sweetener.

Like the essential oil, I like to use Geranium hydrosol to aid in concentration, especially in cases like ADHD, where there's a nervous tension or hyperactivity component. Can be diffused into a private office space during work hours, spritzed over the face before tackling a project, or enjoyed in a glass of water during a meeting or conference call.

As a face toner, this hydrosol is luxurious and sweet on the skin in the morning or the evening prior to applying a face cream. I frequently use the hydrosol as a base for my aqueous skincare formulations, from gels to creams and lotions. It is very soothing to dry, inflamed, and acne-prone skin.

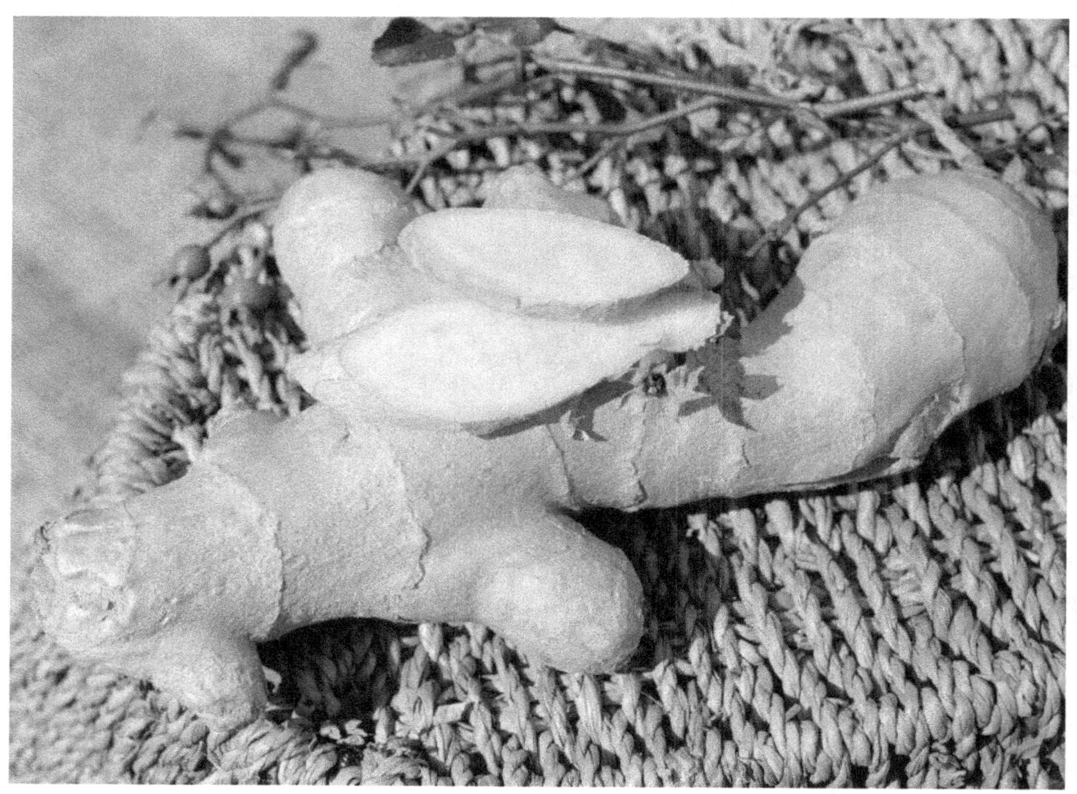

24 GINGER

Ginger is a perennial herb with a knobby, spreading rhizome root system. It was first introduced to the Americans in the 16th century by Francisco de Mendosa, who transplanted it from the East Indies. The herb and essential oil are used for cold conditions like rheumatism and arthritis, as well as for nausea and vomiting.

Common Name(s): Ginger
Botanical Name(s): *Zingiber officinale*
Botanical Family: Zingberaceae (ginger family)
Plant Parts Used: Rhizome (root)
Odor Profile: Pungent, spicy
Flavor: Warm, spicy, pungent, stronger than ginger tea
Safety Considerations: None known
Biophysical Actions: antiemetic, anti-inflammatory, antirheumatic

Ginger is warming and pungent. I love it in the bath on a cold winter's night, spritzed on a knee complaining of the cold weather, or in my nebulizer for sinus congestion due to the common cold. It's a great first-aid tool for morning sickness, motion sickness, following chemotherapy, and other instances of nausea.

Peach-Ginger Agua Fresca

When I lived in Central Mexico, we drank agua fresca of whatever fruit was in season. Free-stone peaches that come a little later in the season are usually easier to remove from their pits, but the first round of peaches are often the juiciest. You can use whichever is in season or grab a bag of frozen peaches at your local market.

1 cup sliced, pitted peaches
1/4 cup fresh lemon juice
4 cups purified water
10 mls ginger hydrosol
honey, to taste

Blend all ingredients in the blender until smooth. Serve at room temperature or chilled.

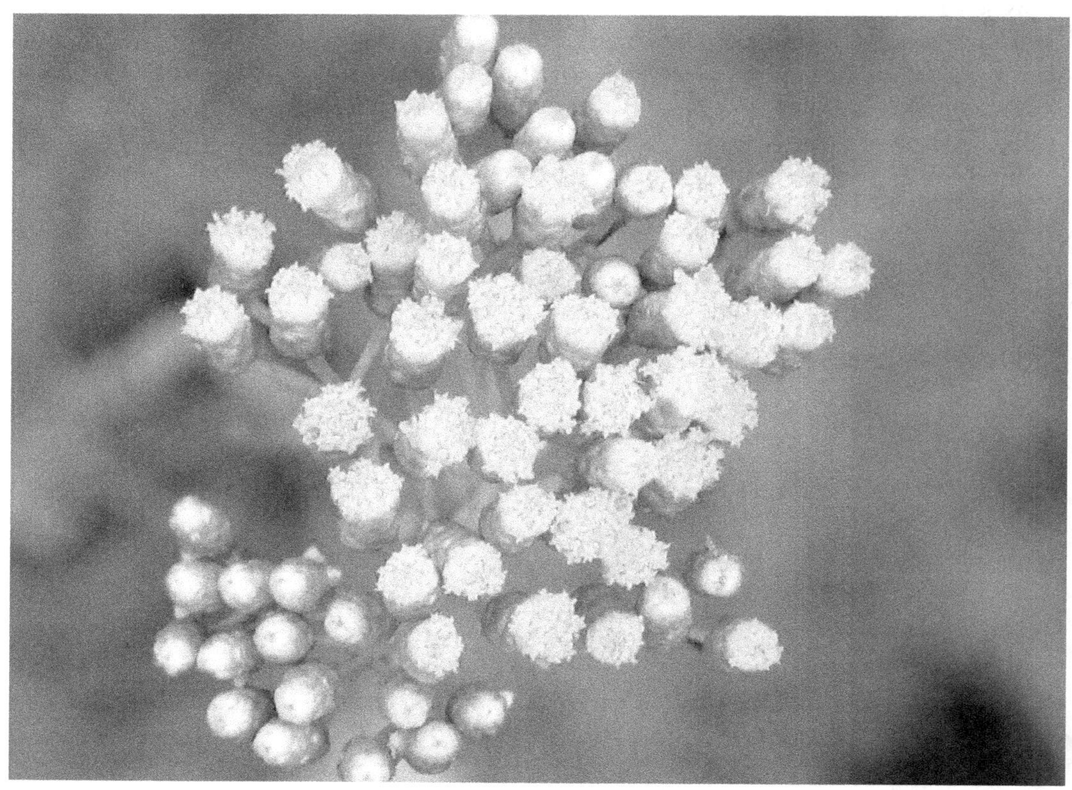

25 HELICHRYSUM

Helichrysum is a strongly aromatic, herbaceous herb that grows to less than a meter (2 feet) in height, with brilliant yellow daisy-like flowers. As of the writing of this monograph, *Helichrysum italicum* is experiencing a higher demand than the market can currently handle, and there have been many adulterated products on the market for a few years now, so buyer beware. Due to this popularity, the essential oil and hydrosol are expensive and it is a bit challenging to find unadulterated sources.

Common Name(s): Helichrysum, Immortelle, Everlasting, Curry Plant
Botanical Name(s): *Helichrusum italicum, Helichrysum angustifolia*
Botanical Family: Asteraceae (daisy family)
Plant Parts Used: Flowering plant
Odor Profile: Earthy herbaceous
Flavor: Bitter earthy herbaceous

Safety Considerations: None known
Biophysical Actions: anticontusion, cicatrisant

While the hydrosol doesn't quite hold a candle to the essential oil's ability to speed up the healing of wounds and contusions, it does have its place. I use it for mild to moderate bruising on unbroken skin to enhance local circulation. For adults, I recommend undiluted for contusions, I spritz it directly on the affected area every few hours, until the pain, swelling, and bruising are resolved, usually 24-48 hours.

I recommend pairing this with German Chamomile for first aid relief of burns, from stovetop to sunburns to radiation burns. It is nice in a warm bath with Ginger for aching joints; and it pairs well with Frankincense as a face toner or gel serum, to reduce the appearance of fine lines and wrinkles.

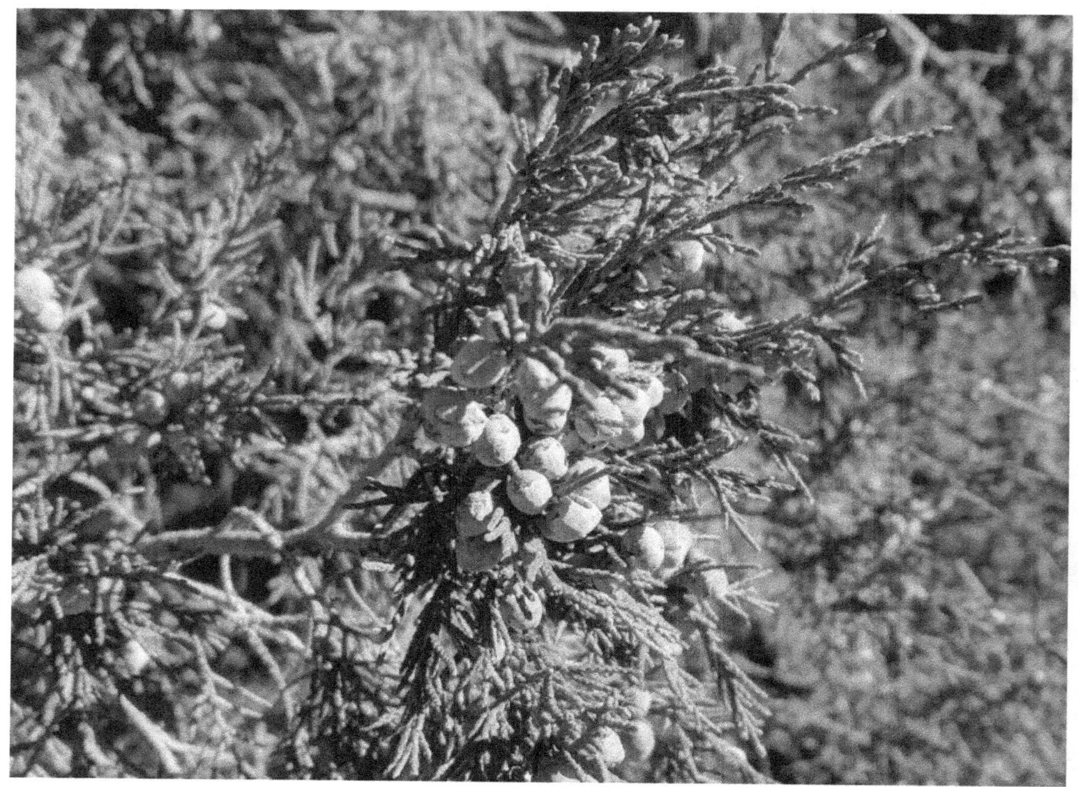

26 JUNIPER BERRY

Juniper is an evergreen tree that reaches 3 meters (9 feet) in height, with wide spreading branches. It has awl-shaped needles with blunt tips that are gray-green to blue-green in color. Immature berries are green and mature berries are a deep purple, it takes 2-3 years for the berries to ripen, and the tree can support both immature and mature berries at the same time.

The berries from the Juniper tree are used to flavor gin, which was originally produced as a medicine to treat stomach complaints, gout, and gallstones as a diuretic.

Common Name(s): Juniper, Common Juniper
Botanical Name(s): *Juniperus communis*

Botanical Family: Cupressaceae (cypress family)
Plant Parts Used: Mature berries
Odor Profile: Sharp, tart, piney with a hint of citrus
Flavor: Bitter piney with a hint of citrus
Safety Considerations: None known
Biophysical Actions: astringent, diuretic, insecticide, urinary antiseptic

My clients tell me this hydrosol tastes like a Christmas or Yule tree. Growing up, our local curendera had us boil the berries in water to make a decoction for stomach viruses. Ever since, I've been a bit squeamish around imbibing gin or the hydrosol, unless it is masked with another flavorant (like the recipe below).

Juniper berry hydrosol's astringent properties and woodsy aroma make it very popular with my male adolescent clients suffering from acne of the face and back. They're quite compliant using it in a spritz as a toner, but I've only gotten a few to successfully use it in a gel or cream. As a urinary antiseptic, I love this in a peri wash at the first sign of a urinary tract infection.

Juniper Watermelon Lemonade

This is a refreshing, non-alcoholic drink that is perfect for gin lovers who want the flavor without the booze.

3 cups lemonade, unsweetened
6-8 cups watermelon, cut into small chunks
1 lemon, sliced into thin rounds for garnish
5-10 mls Juniper Berry hydrosol, to taste

In a blender, puree watermelon -- you may need to do batches, depending on your blender size. Combine lemonade, and pureed watermelon, add 5 mls (1 teaspoon) hydrosol, stir and taste. Add another 5 mls hydrosol if desired. Garnish with lemons. Pairs well with a rocking chair on the back porch.

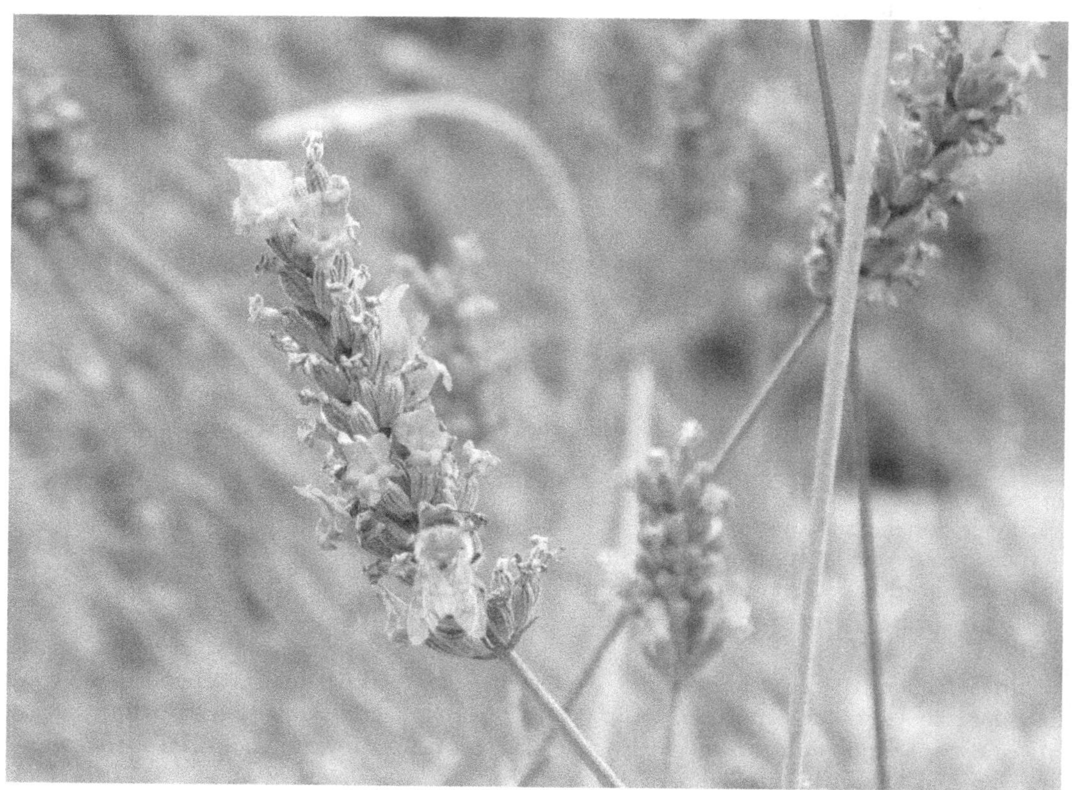

27 LAVENDER

Lavender is an evergreen shrub with pale green, spiky, narrow leaves and purple flowers. The Romans used Lavender to scent their baths, which is how it got its name -- from the Latin word for wash, *lavare*. Culpepper strongly recommended Lavender for 'swooning, fainting, trembling and passions of the heart,' and indicated Lavender hydrosol to 'comfort the stomach.'

Common Name(s): Lavender, French Lavender, True Lavender, English Lavender, Alpine Lavender, Common Lavender
Botanical Name(s): *Lavandula angustifolia, Lavandula officinalis, Lavandula vera*
Botanical Family: Lamiaceae (mint family)
Plant Parts Used: Flowers, leaves, stalks
Odor Profile: Sweet floral with a hint of honey
Flavor: Herbaceous-bitter, floral

Safety Considerations: None known
Biophysical Actions: antispasmodic, anxiolytic, cicatrisant, relaxant, sedative

Another first aid-in-a-bottle hydrosol. Lavender is soothing, sedating and an overall good choice for pediatrics. Use it topically for sunburns, cuts, insect bites, heat rashes, and to cool the skin as a face toner. Or add it to water or milk (dairy or non) to relax and calm in a bedtime drink.

Lavender Hot Cocoa

I love a cup of cocoa in the evenings; I paired it with lavender hydrosol once and was smitten!

1 ounce roughly chopped dark chocolate
3/4 cup milk (dairy or non)
honey, to taste
5 mls lavender hydrosol

In a small saucepan heat the milk and chocolate over medium until the chocolate dissolves. Remove from heat, stir in lavender hydrosol and honey and serve.

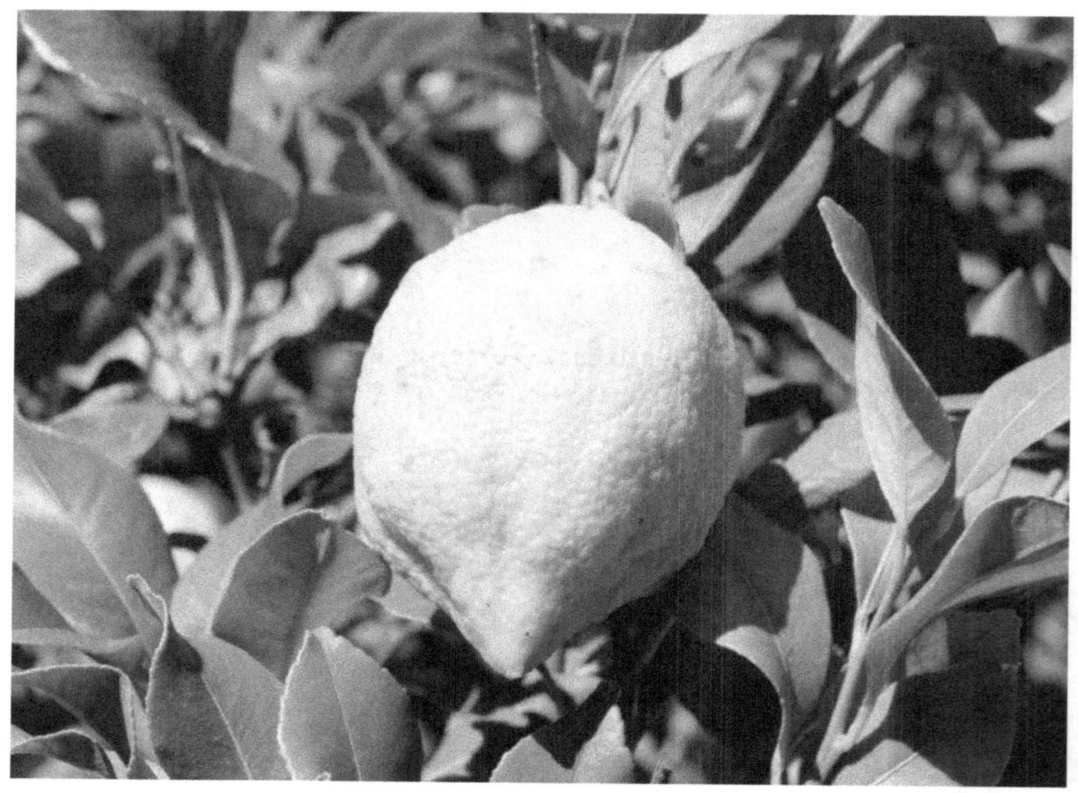

28 LEMON

Lemon trees originated in Asia and can grow up to 6 meters (20 feet) in height, with dark green serrated leaves and highly fragrant flowers. They grow well in the Mediterranean and the United States, in Florida and California. The essential oil is obtained from grating and pressing the outer peel of the mature fruits. The hydrosol is steam distilled and has a subtler aroma profile.

Common Name(s): Lemon
Botanical Name(s): *Citrus limon, Citrus limonum*
Botanical Family: Rutaceae (citrus family)
Plant Parts Used: Whole fruit and/or rind
Odor Profile: Citrusy
Flavor: Bitter citrusy
Safety Considerations: None known. Due to the steam distillation, the hydrosol is not

phototoxic, while the cold-pressed essential oil is
Biophysical Actions: antiseptic, astringent, cicatrisant, depurative, diuretic, tonic

Lemon hydrosol is a great tool for skin that is dull, oily, and congested. It can be used at full strength for especially challenging skin conditions or diluted in half with another complementary hydrosol. While not as stimulating and uplifting as the essential oil, the hydrosol is a gentler remedy for mental fatigue and lack of concentration. Lemon hydrosol is a good choice for nebulizer use in wellness plans for asthma, bronchitis, and respiratory health. My clients enjoy this hydrosol in their nebulizer in the weeks and months after quitting cigarettes.

Warm Lemon-Rosemary Green Bean Salad

This salad is a perfect side dish when green beans are at their peak, it's also pretty tasty if you can only get your hands on frozen green beans.

1 pound summer beans – green, purple, yellow, or mixed
2 tablespoons olive oil
1 tablespoon vinegar, such as white wine or apple cider
1 teaspoon lemon hydrosol
1 teaspoon rosemary hydrosol
1 garlic clove, minced
salt and pepper, freshly ground
1/4 cup sliced almonds

Place the almonds in a skillet and toast until browned and fragrant. Remove from heat and cool. Bring 2 quarts of salted water to a boil. Meanwhile, wash and trim beans. Boil beans for 3-4 minutes or until crisp-tender, drain immediately and plunge into an iced water bath. In a serving bowl, whisk together garlic, olive oil, vinegar, hydrosols, salt and pepper until well combined. Toss beans with vinaigrette and let sit for a few minutes. Just before serving, add toasted almonds.

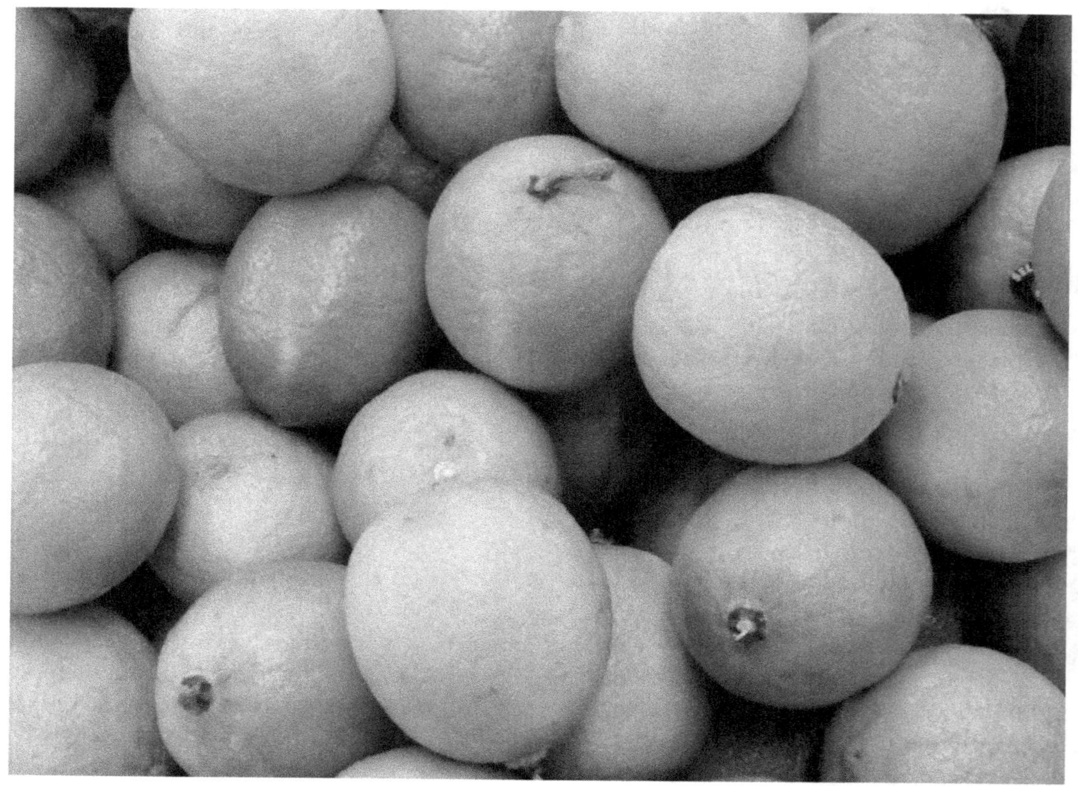

29 LIME

Known as the Key Lime, Mexican Lime, and Bartender's Lime, this lime tree grows up to 5 meters (16 feet), with green ovate leaves and small yellowish-white flowers with a slight purple tinge on the margins.

We grow this lime here in Texas, so I'm lucky to have fresh, ripe fruit available year-round to go into my limeade or into the still for a hydrosol.

Common Name(s): Lime
Botanical Name(s): *Citrus aurantifolia*
Botanical Family: Rutaceae (citrus family)
Plant Parts Used: Whole fruit and/or rind
Odor Profile: Super sweet citrusy, it smells like candied limes
Flavor: Bitter citrusy

Safety Considerations: Due to the steam distillation, the hydrosol is not phototoxic, while the cold-pressed essential oil is
Biophysical Actions: antiseptic, astringent, cicatrisant, depurative, diuretic, tonic

Similar to usage of the lemon, this one just has a much sweeter aroma and tends to be more popular for some. I give clients the choice of their preference when I have both hydrosols in stock. One of my clients swears by her Lime hydrosol during the summer months for her hot, throbbing varicose veins.

Lime-Cilantro Nice Cream

This is my favorite ice cream recipe of all time and I've made it with a ton of variations. That sweet-tart lime hydrosol contrasted with the spicy-herbaceous cilantro is a great flavor, but you can use other herbs and hydrosols in the recipe base to make a combination you love. Cinnamon hydrosol and rum soaked raisins are pretty stellar here too.

2 cans coconut milk
2 tablespoons arrowroot powder
1/2 cup sugar
1 teaspoon vanilla extract
15 mls Lime hydrosol
1 teaspoon finely chopped cilantro (coriander leaves)

In a small bowl, whisk 1/4 cup coconut milk with arrowroot powder until smooth. Add remaining coconut milk and sugar to a medium-sized saucepan and heat over medium-high until simmering. Stir in arrowroot coconut milk, and whisk constantly. Coconut milk will thicken within a few minutes. Remove from heat. Stir in vanilla, hydrosol, and chopped cilantro. Chill for several hours in the refrigerator. Proceed to freeze using an ice cream machine, following manufacturer's instructions. Serve.

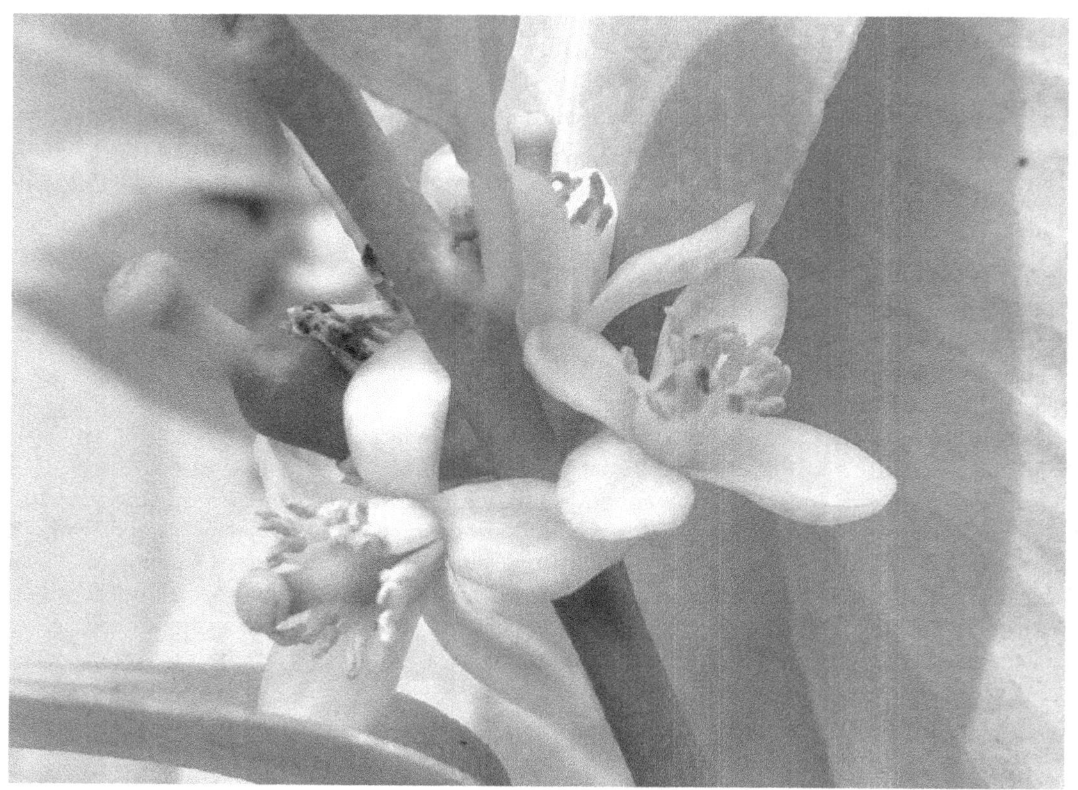

30 NEROLI

Neroli is the blossom from the Bitter Orange tree native to Southeast Asia, but now growing in the wild around the globe in temperate climates. The Seville bitter orange tree is used to make marmalades. The hydrosol has a long history of flavoring and perfuming bitter herbs and medicines that were taken in syrup or liquid form by mouth.

Neroli is an intensely floral aroma and the hydrosol is a much gentler way to enjoy the scent for those who find the essential oil overpowering.

Common Name(s): Neroli (Bitter Orange Blossom)
Botanical Name(s): *Citrus aurantium*
Botanical Family: Rutaceae (citrus family)
Plant Parts Used: Flowers

Odor Profile: Intense floral with slight citrus notes
Flavor: Sweet-floral
Safety Considerations: None known. My clients with multiple chemical sensitivities and floral scent aversion find the hydrosol easier to tolerate than the essential oil.
Biophysical Actions: antidepressant, anxiolytic, relaxant, sedative

The essential oil is used for shock, acute stress, panic attacks, and insomnia resulting from high stress. I use the hydrosol for mild cases of anxiety, panic, acute stress, depression, and seasonal affective disorder. In times of political unrest, environmental disasters, and terrorist attacks, I can't keep the hydrosol in stock.

Neroli hydrosol is also nice in cosmetic applications for dry, irritated, sensitive, and mature skin types. The heady aroma usually serves as the only scent I wear on a night out with friends, to a party, or a wedding.

Mauresque Cocktail - an Aperitif

2 ounces pastis (recipe follows)
1 ounce orgeat syrup (recipe follows)
Sparkling water to taste
Stir pastis and orgeat syrup together into an old fashioned glass. Add sparkling water and enjoy before dinner.

To make pastis:

8 star anise pods
1 heaping tablespoon licorice root
1 scant teaspoon fennel seeds
1/2 teaspoon whole coriander seeds
1 scant teaspoon anise seeds
4-6 pippali peppers (available at most Indian markets)

Place all in the blender or food processor until roughly chopped. Pour into a pint-sized mason jar and fill with 1-1/2 cups vodka. Shake daily for one week. Strain. Make a simple syrup of 1/2 cup sugar and 1/2 cup water. Combine simple syrup and pastis in a quart mason jar.

To make orgeat:

2 cups raw pecans, macadamia, almonds, or walnuts
1-1/2 cups sugar
1-1/2 cups water
30-60 mls neroli hydrosol

Heat chosen nuts in a skillet until fragrant and slightly browned. Let cool. Transfer to blender or food processor and pulverize until pieces are pea-sized or smaller. Add to a saucepan with sugar and water, bring to a simmer, and stir until sugar is dissolved. Remove from heat and let steep for 3-4 hours or overnight. Strain through cheesecloth. Add hydrosol and refrigerate.

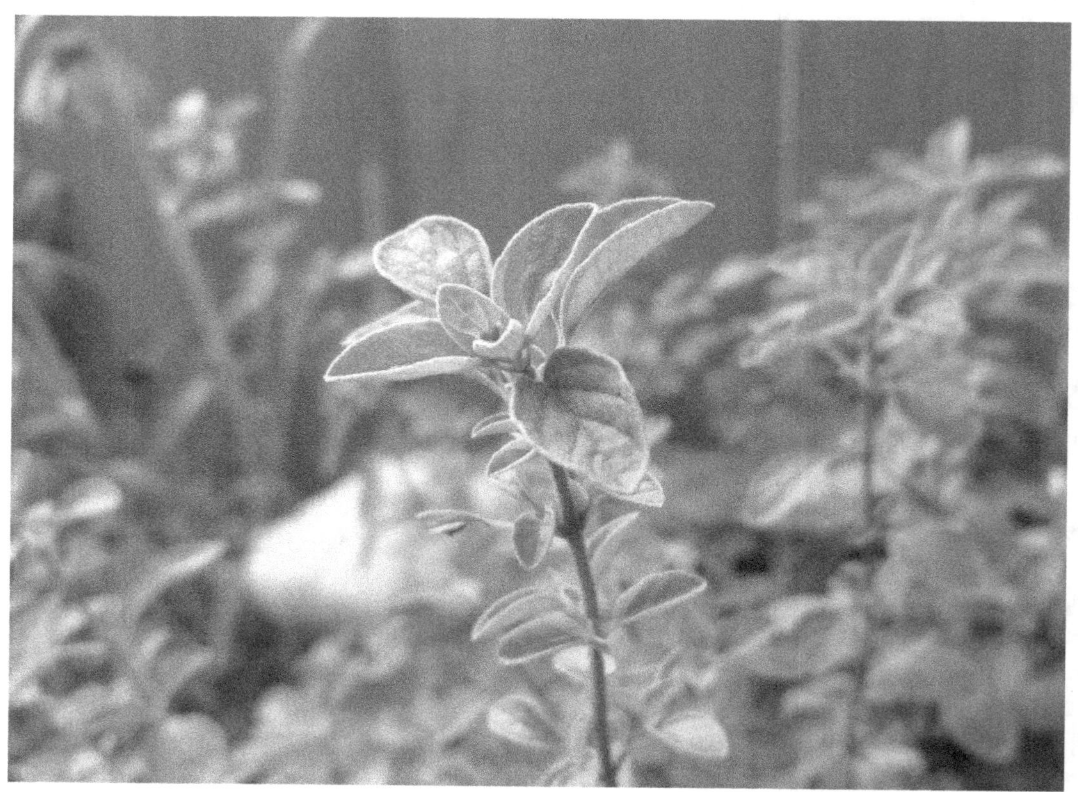

31 OREGANO

Oregano is an aromatic, woody-based perennial herb that grows up to 1 meter (3 feet) in height, and has ovate shaped green leaves with white to purplish flowers. It is native to the Mediterranean, Europe, South and Central Asia, and is cultivated around the globe.

Common Name(s): Oregano
Botanical Name(s): *Origanum vulgare*
Botanical Family: Lamiaceae (mint family)
Plant Parts Used: Aerial parts of flowering plant
Odor Profile: Spicy herbaceous
Flavor: Warm spicy herbaceous
Safety Considerations: The essential oil is a mucous membrane irritant and I have found the hydrosol is better tolerated when diluted

Biophysical Actions: antifungal, anti-infectious, antimicrobial

Oregano hydrosol is one of our strongest antimicrobial hydrosols and a much safer option to using the essential oil. Here in Texas, we have a nasty problem with airborne mold year-round, resulting in chronic sinusitis and acute fungal sinus infections that can't be touched with antibiotics. I recommend 5mls of the hydrosol in a nasal rinse for year-round residents.

For culinary use, the hydrosol is delicious added to pizza and spaghetti sauces after cooking, and to flavor salads, warm and cold vegetable dishes, and soups.

Perineal Hydrosol Rinse

A hydrosol rinse of the perineum may be desired for several reasons:
- Urinary Tract Infection – at the first sign of suspected symptoms.
- Following Intercourse – an antimicrobial rinse may be desired to prevent a UTI, vaginitis, or a yeast infection after swapping microbes with an existing or new sexual partner. Or for those who have a tendency to get cystitis or urinary tract infections following sex.
- Vaginitis – at the first sign of suspected symptoms
- Postpartum or following minor perineal surgery – switch out the antimicrobial hydrosols for soothing Lavender, Chamomile, Cucumber, or Rose to help heal tissue and decrease discomfort.

10 mls antimicrobial hydrosol – choose from Tea Tree, Oregano, or Thyme hydrosols
5 mls Lavender hydrosol
Filtered water

In a 3-ounce squeeze bottle, combine the two hydrosols and top off with filtered water. Shake to mix well. To use: Squirt the urethra and perineum with the hydrosol rinse. This rinse can be used before and after sex, or at the first signs of a UTI or vaginitis, and subsequently after each urination, until the symptoms have improved. Keep in mind that UTIs can lead to kidney issues and should be monitored by your medical professional, especially when accompanied with low back pain.

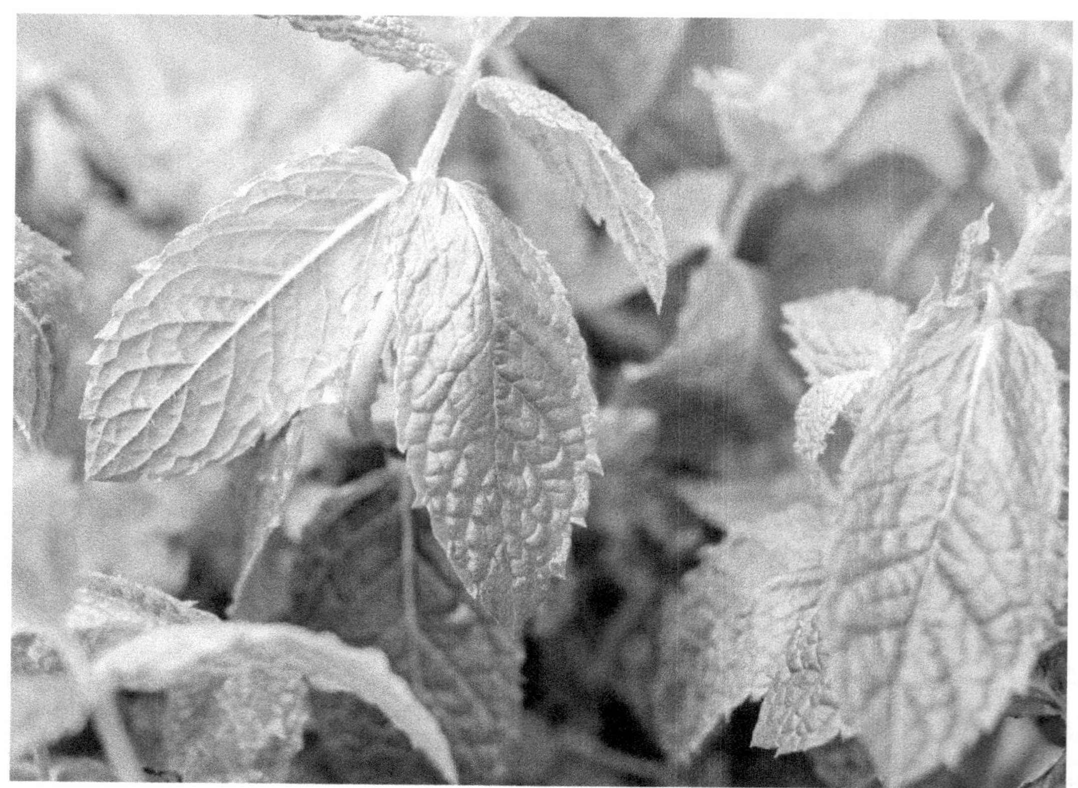

32 PEPPERMINT

Peppermint is a naturally-occurring hybrid of *Mentha spicata* (Spearmint) and *Mentha aquatic* (Watermint). It is an aromatic perennial herb that grows from 30-90 centimeters (12-35 inches) in height, with wide-spreading rhizomes. The leaves are dark green with reddish veins and purple flowers. It has a long history of use from ancient Egyptians, Romans, and Greeks, and was added to the *London Pharmacopoeia* in 1721.

Common Name(s): Peppermint, Mint, Balm Mint, Brandy Mint
Botanical Name(s): *Menth x piperita*
Botanical Family: Lamiaceae (mint family)
Plant Parts Used: Leaves and flowering tops
Odor Profile: Sweet menthol minty
Flavor: Sweet menthol minty

Safety Considerations: None known. The essential oil is a mucous membrane irritant
Biophysical Actions: analgesic, carminative, cephalic, decongestant, stomachic

Peppermint hydrosol is nice first aid option for bug bites that are hot and itchy, for relief from jet lag, and spritzed on the legs after strenuous activities in the heat of summer. Sipping on a glass of water with peppermint hydrosol added has been helpful for some of my clients with morning sickness, while ginger, cardamom, and lemon were better fits for others. It can be used in the nebulizer or nasal rinse for sinus congestion and paired with a stronger antimicrobial hydrosol for sinus infections. Peppermint's tropism is for the stomach and upper digestive tract and it is useful as a digestive aid taken in water before a meal or in the event of a headache caused by overeating.

Aromatic Foot or Hand Soak

We know that essential oils and water don't mix, but hydrosols sure do! Soaking the feet after a long day of walking or standing is complete bliss. A hand soak can feel great on arthritic joints, chilblains in the winter, and gardener's hands in the summer.

10-40 mls hydrosols – Lavender (to ease aching feet or hands), Peppermint (to ease hot, tired feet), Lemon (to ease hot or odorous feet)
1/4-1/2 cup soaking salts – Epsom's, Himalayan pink, Dead Sea

Fill a basin large enough for your hands or feet half way with warm water. Avoid using too hot water, so the skin isn't scalded or damaged. Pour your hydrosol(s) and salts into the warm water, and stir with your hand to dissolve.

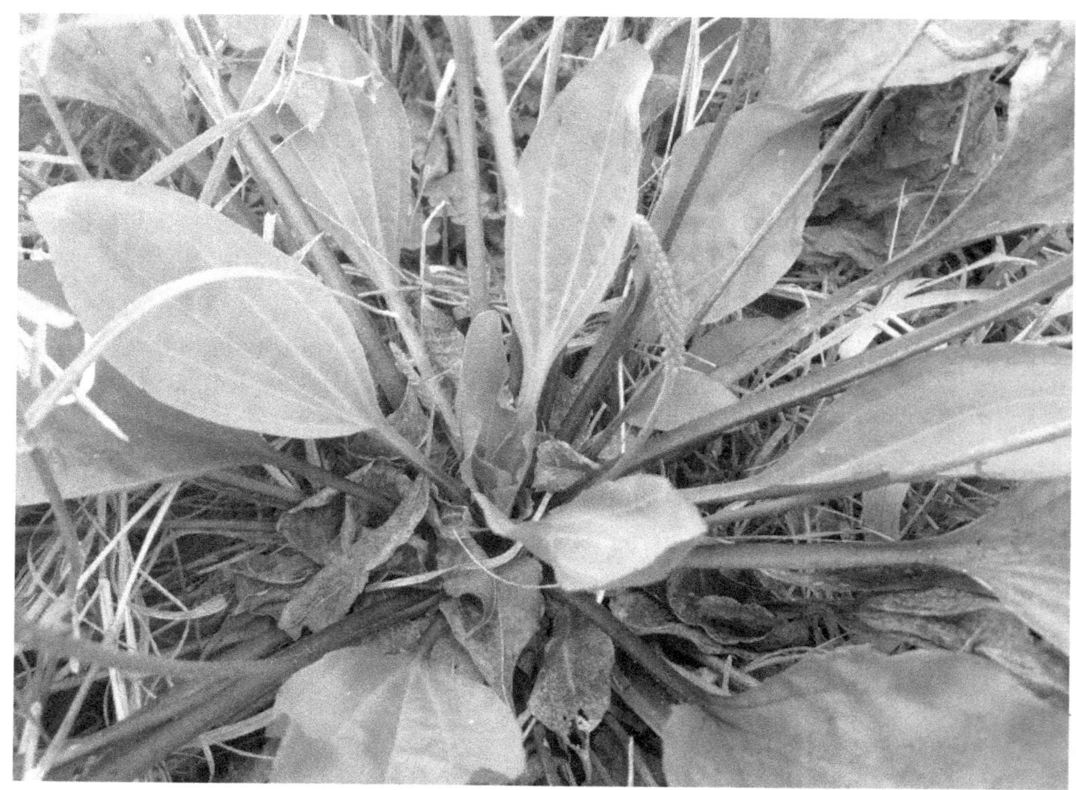

33 PLANTAIN

Plantain is an herbaceous perennial plant with oval shaped leaves and flowers that appear in dense spikes. The herb is traditionally used for wounds, sores, stings, and bites.

Common Name(s): Plantain
Botanical Name(s): *Plantago major*
Botanical Family: Plantaginaeae (plantain family)
Plant Parts Used: Leaves
Odor Profile: Light herbaceous
Flavor: Gently herbaceous
Safety Considerations: None known.
Biophysical Actions: analgesic, antimicrobial, cicatrisant

Plantain hydrosol isn't nearly as good as having the fresh plant on hand, but I keep it in my first aid repertoire when the frost has pushed the plant back into the ground for the season. Grieve notes, 'The distilled water with a little alum and honey dissolved in it is of good use for washing, cleansing and healing a sore ulcerated mouth or throat' Salmon's Herbal, 1710 (Grieve 1992). Plantain hydrosol has a light green aroma, and I like to use it on the skin after a cut, scrape, or bug bite. It's also useful in an oral rinse for inflamed gums, a burned tongue, or sore throat from postnasal drip during allergy season.

Mouthwash

15 mls Frankincense-Myrrh resin extract
15 mls Lemon Balm extract
3 ounces Plantain hydrosol
1 ounce Peppermint, Cinnamon, or Fragonia™ hydrosol

To make the Frankincense-Myrrh extract: add 1 part resins to a mason jar with 5 parts high-proof alcohol. Shake daily for a minimum of 2 weeks. Strain using muslin or an unbleached paper towel.

To make the Lemon Balm extract: add 1 part dried Lemon Balm leaves to a mason jar with 5 parts high-proof alcohol. Shake daily for a minimum of 2 weeks. Strain using muslin or a fine-mesh strainer.

Combine the extracts and hydrosol(s) in a pint-sized mason jar and shake well to combine. Use 30-60 mls as a mouth rinse or gargle. For a child-friendly formula, try spearmint and chamomile hydrosols diluted 1:4 (1 part hydrosol to 4 parts water) with a few drops of vegetable glycerin to sweeten it.

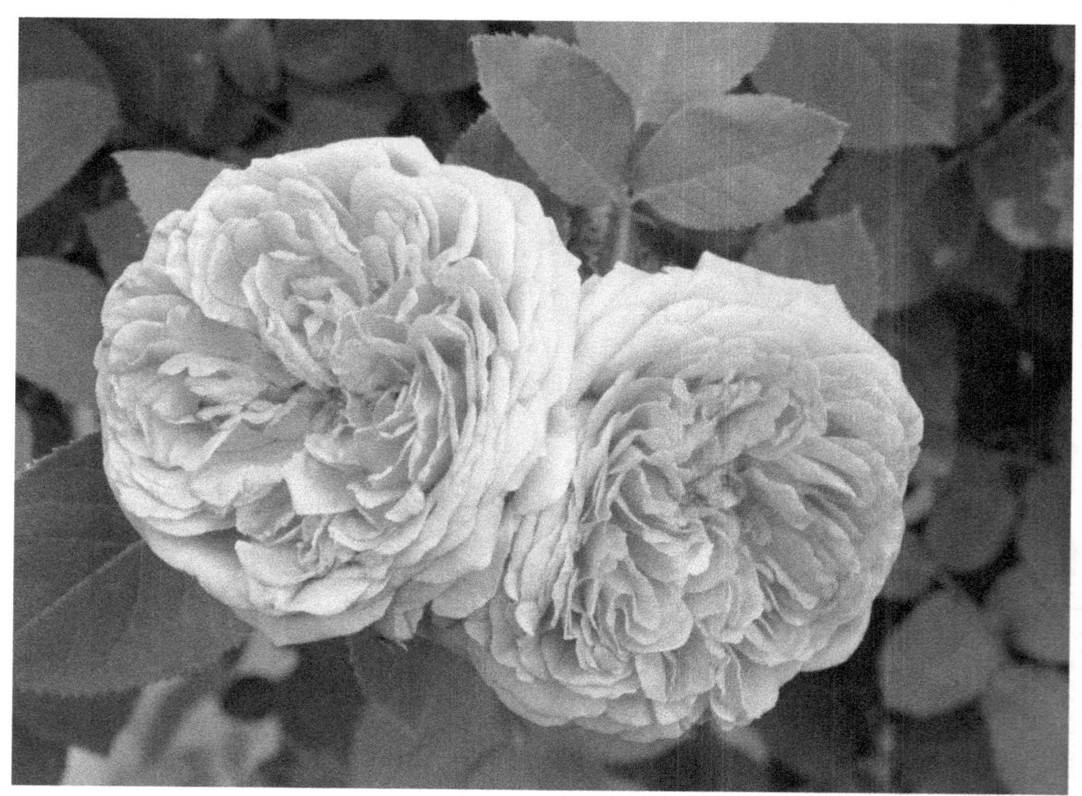

34 ROSE

Damask rose is a deciduous shrub reaching over 2 meters (7 feet) in height, with green pinnate leaves and medium pink to light red flowers. This variety of rose is used for its absolute, essential oil, hydrosol, fresh flowers, for culinary practices around the globe, and dried flowers, as an herbal tea.

Common Name(s): Damask Rose, Bulgarian Rose
Botanical Name(s): *Rosa damascena*
Botanical Family: Rosaceae (rose family)
Plant Parts Used: Flowers
Odor Profile: Sweet strongly floral
Flavor: Sweet floral
Safety Considerations: None known.

Biophysical Actions: anxiolytic, antidepressant, aphrodisiac, calming

A lot of the commercially available Rose hydrosol on the market is what we consider biowaste in the industry. A byproduct of distillation for essential oils. Seek out an artisan distiller that distills Rose for its hydrosol alone.

Rose hydrosol is gently cooling, making it a popular choice for inflamed skin conditions like eczema, psoriasis, and acne. In a glass of water, it can ease feelings of anxiousness and mild depression, it pairs well with talk therapy sessions, as well as massage and reflexology sessions to support relaxation methods, and is used well afterwards, to recall those sensations of harmony of mind, body, and spirit.

Rose water has a lengthy history of use in culinary recipes, from sorbets to Turkish delight, and candied borage flowers.

Honeyed Figs with Rose Whipped Cream

If you've made up a batch of Rose-Tulsi Cordial you can use it in this recipe in place of the brandy and honey.

1 cup dried figs
1 cup brandy
2 tablespoons honey

Macerate figs in brandy and honey overnight. Remove the figs and slice in half, lengthwise. Gently simmer on the stovetop in the brandy-honey juice adding another 1/4 cup honey and 1/4 cup water. Reduce liquid to half, remove from heat and cool for 5 minutes. Serve in shallow bowls with a dollop of:

Rose Whipped Cream

Infusing whipped cream with hydrosols is a simple way to really jazz up a dessert. I use rose whipped cream in fruit parfait cups, over cobblers and pies, and the occasional breakfast waffle for Jazz Sundays at our casa.

1/2 cup heavy cream
5 mls rose hydrosol
confectioners' sugar, to taste

Using a whisk attachment in a blender, whip the cream and hydrosol until soft peaks form. Add the sugar; whip to combine.

You can also make aromatic whipped creams with cinnamon to top your slice of pecan pie, with sweet orange for a raspberry parfait cup, or neroli to scoop onto your peach cobbler.

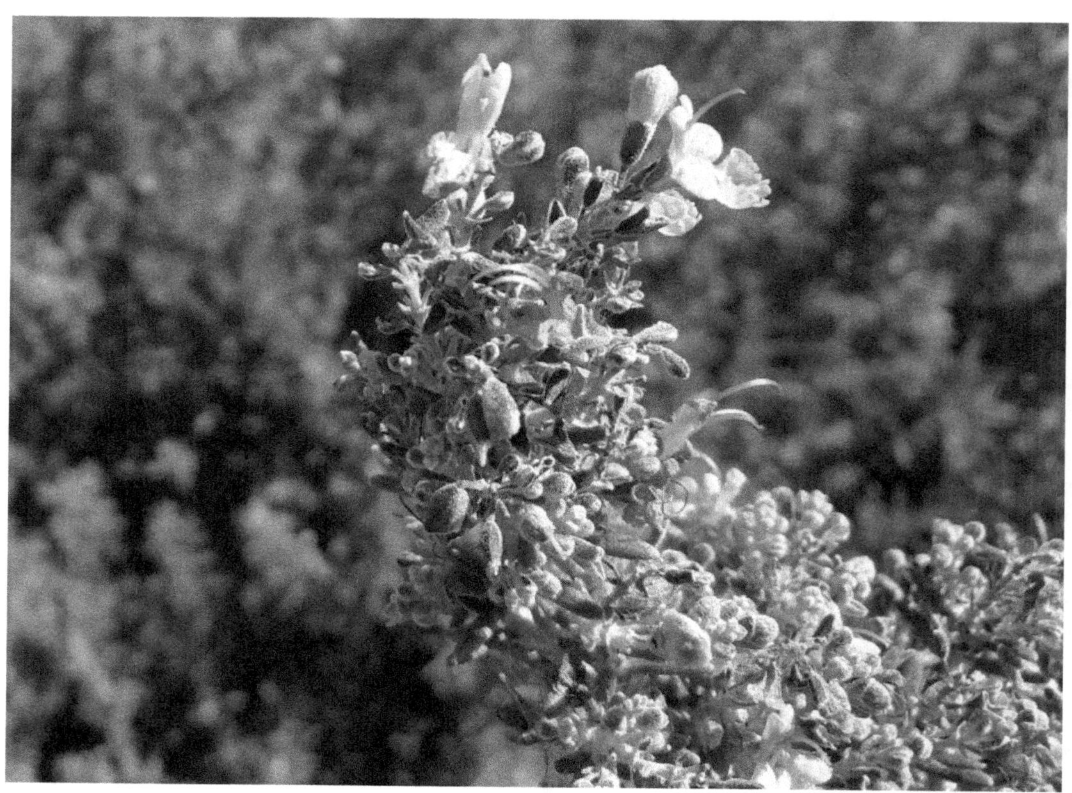

35 ROSEMARY

Rosemary is an aromatic shrub that grows up to 2 meters (6 feet) in height, with silvery-green, needle-shaped leaves, and pale blue flowers. Rosemary has several chemo-types available: camphor, cineole, verbenone, and borneol. Cineole is popular for upper respiratory issues (Moroccan, Tunisian). Verbenone is indicated for skin blends. Borneol is high in alcohols and indicated for more general use (France). Camphor chemotype has up to 30% camphor and is used with caution. Rosemary gets its name from the Latin *ros-marinus*, meaning sea-dew, referring to its natural habitat. The hydrosol is referred to as the *Dew of Rosemary*. The Spanish believed the rosemary bush sheltered the Virgin Mary in the flight to Egypt. Greek students put sprigs of rosemary in their hair to aid in concentration during exams. In Asia, rosemary is planted on graves to invoke the guidance of the deceased for the living.

Common Name(s): Rosemary, Compass plant
Botanical Name(s): *Rosmarinus officinalis, Rosmarinus coronarium*
Botanical Family: Lamiaceae (mint family)
Plant Parts Used: Flowering tops and leaves
Odor Profile: Pungent herbaceous
Flavor: Bitter herbaceous
Safety Considerations: None known.
Biophysical Actions: antimicrobial, cephalic, expectorant, stimulant (mental and circulatory)

Like the essential oil, Rosemary chemotypes indicate different usage based on potential chemistry. **Camphoraceous** and **Cineole-rich** Rosemary chemotype hydrosols would be used for their expectorant and mucalytic actions in a nebulizer, in hair rinses or sprays for hair growth and scalp stimulation, and, in oral doses, as an antispasmodic for intestinal cramping. **Verbenone** is a shoe-in for cosmetic formulations to nurture environmentally damaged, aging, and acneic skin. Verbenone is also a lovely choice for the parasympathetic nervous system and can be used in the evening without disrupting sleep like the Camphor or Cineole CTs.

Rosemary-Berry Syrup

4 cups water
1 cup fresh or frozen mixed berries
½ cup dried hawthorn berries
¼ cup dried goji berries
¼ cup fresh rosemary
10 mls (2 teaspoons) rosemary hydrosol, to taste
1 cup honey, to taste

Simmer water, berries, and fresh rosemary for 30-45 minutes to reduce by half. Cool slightly then strain using fine mesh sieve. When cooled somewhat, stir in honey and hydrosol, tasting at intervals, until desired flavor is achieved. Makes a great cocktail or mocktail base, can be drizzled over oatmeal or ice cream, or used in dressings and marinades.

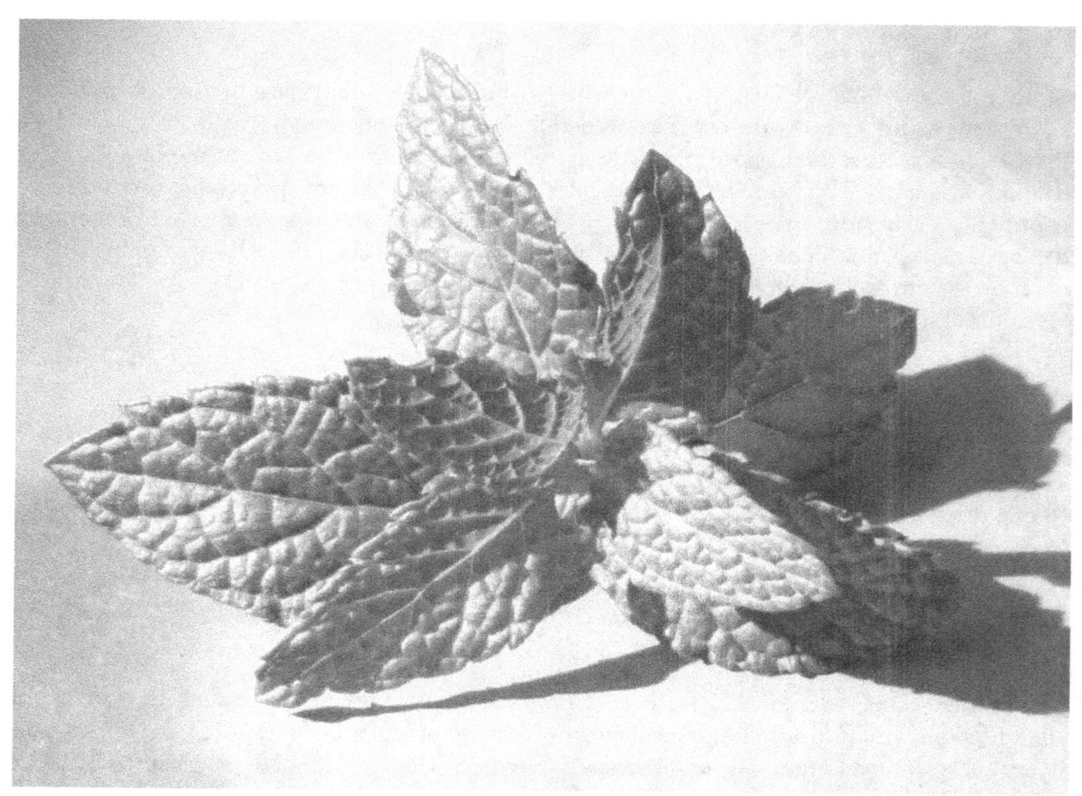

36 SPEARMINT

Spearmint is an herbaceous, rhizomatous, perennial plant, growing up to 1 meter (3 feet) in height, with green leaves and pink or white flowers, native to much of Europe and Asia. It has been naturalized in North and South America as well as parts of Northern and Western Africa.

Common Name(s): Spearmint
Botanical Name(s): *Mentha spicata, Mentha cardiaca*
Botanical Family: Lamiaceae (mint family)
Plant Parts Used: Flowering tops and leaves
Odor Profile: Sweet minty with a hint of citrus
Flavor: Sweet mint
Safety Considerations: None known.

Biophysical Actions: anodyne, antiemetic, antispasmodic, carminative, stomachic

Sweet-green spearmint is calming and used for flatulence and indigestion (Grieve 1992), making it a great choice for an after dinner digestif. For infants with colic, a warm bath with 5 mls of the hydrosol can be soothing and comforting. Use orally for older children with nausea or after vomiting, to soothe the digestive system and aid in restorative sleep.

Electrolyte Formula

Useful after diarrhea, fevers, heat exhaustion, vomiting, or a period of strenuous physical activity producing excessive sweating.

15 mls (1 tablespoon) hydrosol - Spearmint, Peppermint, Chamomile, Lavender, Thyme, Lemon Balm
1 quart filtered water
½ teaspoon high-quality salt
½ teaspoon baking soda
30-45 mls (2-3 tablespoons) honey, sugar, or maple syrup

In a quart mason jar, combine salt, baking soda, honey, hydrosol, and a few ounces of filtered water. Seal and shake to dissolve the honey and salt. Fill remainder of jar with filtered water. Serve 2-4 ounces at a time and sip slowly.

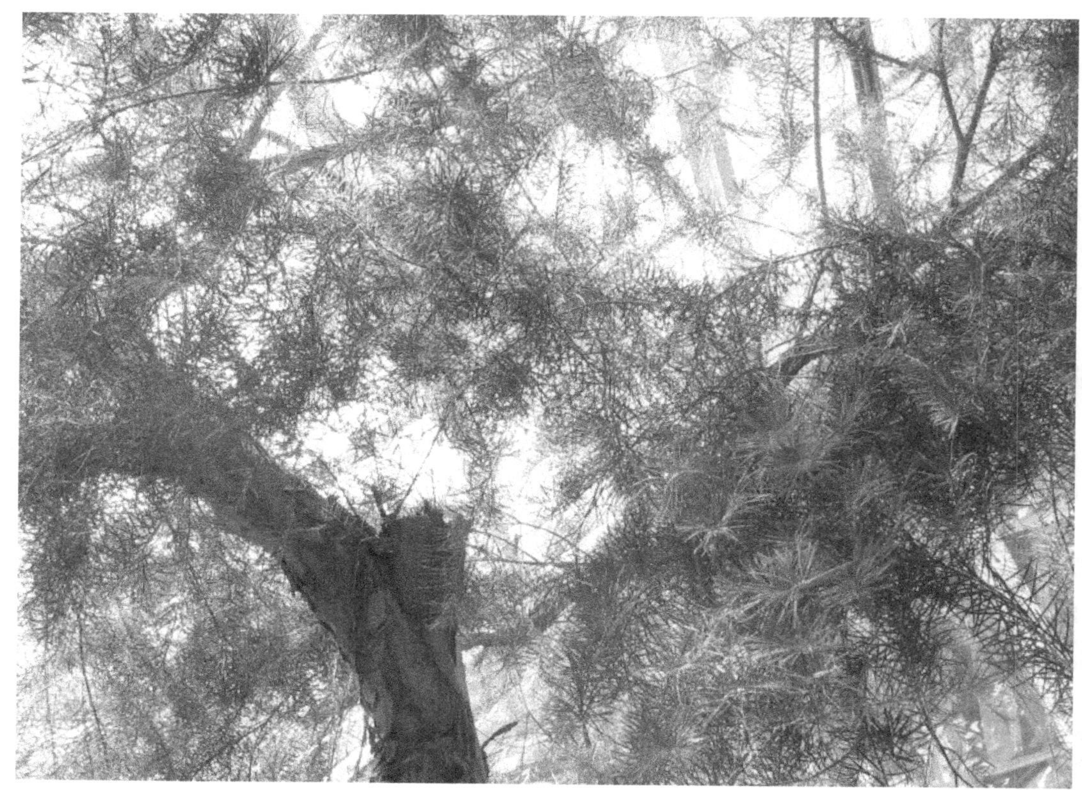

37 TEA TREE

Tea Tree is a small tree growing to 7 meters (20 feet) in height, with papery bark, smooth leaves, and white or off-white flowers appearing in a mass of stamen spikes. Tea tree is the general name for the Melaleuca, Leptospermum, Kunzea, and Baeckea genus. Aborigines have used Tea Tree against infection for hundreds of years, taking it internally as a tea and externally as a poultice on wounds.

Common Name(s): Tea Tree, Narrow-Leaved Paperbark, Narrow-Leaved Ti Tree
Botanical Name(s): *Melaleuca alternifolia*
Botanical Family: Myrtaceae (myrtle family)
Plant Parts Used: Leaves and twigs
Odor Profile: Medicinal pungent
Flavor: Bitter medicinal

Safety Considerations: None known.
Biophysical Actions: antibacterial, antifungal, antimicrobial, antiseptic, antiviral, bactericidal, cicatrisant, immunostimulant

Tea Tree hydrosol isn't as strong as the essential oil, but I prefer to have it on hand for washing of wounds, cuts, scrapes, and for fungal infections like Athlete's foot and ringworm. It's got a very strong medicinal smell, which makes it less popular than some of the other antimicrobial hydrosol options. Consider it in respiratory wellness plans for chest and sinus infections in the nebulizer.

Drawing Clay

Drawing clays can be used to gently draw out a foreign object, poison, or infection from a small skin wound. I use drawing clays for insect bites and stings, stubborn splinters in a finger or foot, or a small cut that needs to be drained of pus.

1 teaspoon clay
enough hydrosol to form a thick paste

Apply a nickel- or dime-sized amount of the clay to the affected area. You can cover it with a bandage to prevent it from flaking off during your activities over the next hour or so. Repeat as needed.

Herbalist Stephen Harrod Buhner recommends using a drawing clay with andrographis (*Andrographis paniculata*) alcohol extract on a tick bite -- after the tick has been removed -- to prevent an active infection. I recommend adding the andrographis extract to the above formula, in equal parts with your selected hydrosol. Hydrosols that would be appropriate would include Thyme, Oregano, Tea Tree, and Fragonia™.

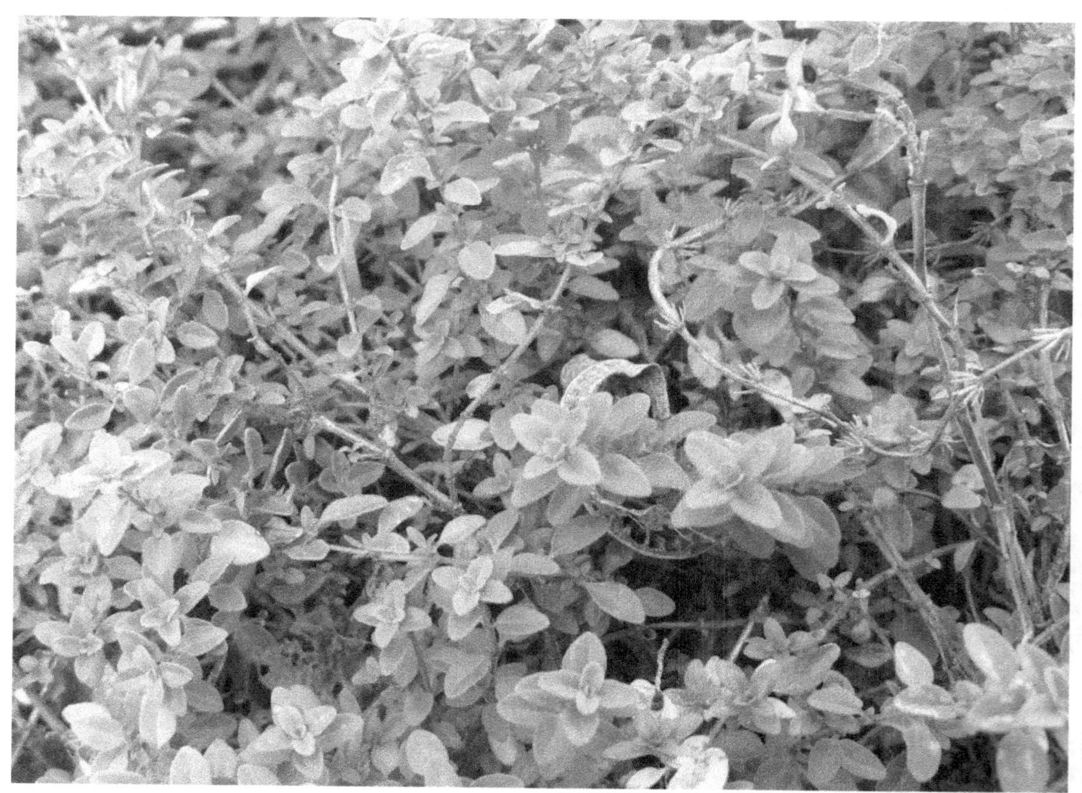

38 THYME

Thyme is an herbaceous, woody-based, perennial, growing up to 30 centimeters (1 foot) in height and spread with aromatic grey-green leaves and clusters of pink to purple flowers native to Southern Europe and the Mediterranean.

Common Name(s): Thyme, German Thyme, Garden Thyme, Common Thyme
Botanical Name(s): *Thymus vulgaris*
Botanical Family: Lamiaceae (mint family)
Plant Parts Used: Aerial parts
Odor Profile: Spicy herbaceous green
Flavor: Spicy, warming herbaceous
Safety Considerations: None known.
Biophysical Actions: antibacterial, antifungal, antimicrobial, antiseptic, antiviral,

bactericidal, cicatrisant, immunostimulant

Like the essential oil, Thyme chemotypes indicate different usage based on potential chemistry. **Carvacrol and Thymol/Carvacrol Chemotypes**: The hydrosols obtained from these chemotypes are used as antiseptics in oral care for sore throats, mouth ulcers, gingivitis, and tooth abscesses (Catty 2001, Grieve 1998). It's also used for insect bites, acne (Price & Price 1999), dermatitis, eczema (Rose 1999), and to revitalize the hair and scalp (Grosjean 1993). **Sweet Thyme – Linalool, Geraniol, and Thujanol Chemotypes**: The hydrosols obtained from the Sweet Thyme chemotypes are used as rinses for eye infections (Price & Price 1999), at 50%, as a digestive tonic (Catty 2001), and as an antifungal against Candida albicans.

Strawberry-Thyme Lassi – a Yogurt Drink

With origins in India, this fermented beverage is delicious paired with your favorite curry.

2 cups whole milk or coconut yogurt
1 cup fresh strawberries
1/2 cup water
honey, to taste
5-10 mls (1-2 teaspoons) thyme hydrosol

In a blender, puree all ingredients until smooth. Chill for an hour, then serve.

I make lassis throughout the year; in addition to Strawberry and Thyme I've found some other delightful hydrosol + fruit combinations:

Peaches + Basil hydrosol
Mango + Cardamom hydrosol
Mixed berries + Rosemary hydrosol
Pineapple + Ginger hydrosol
Bananas + Neroli hydrosol
Cooked, peeled beets + Ginger & Mint hydrosols
Avocado + Rose hydrosol
Kiwi + Fennel hydrosol
Cantaloupe + Cinnamon hydrosol

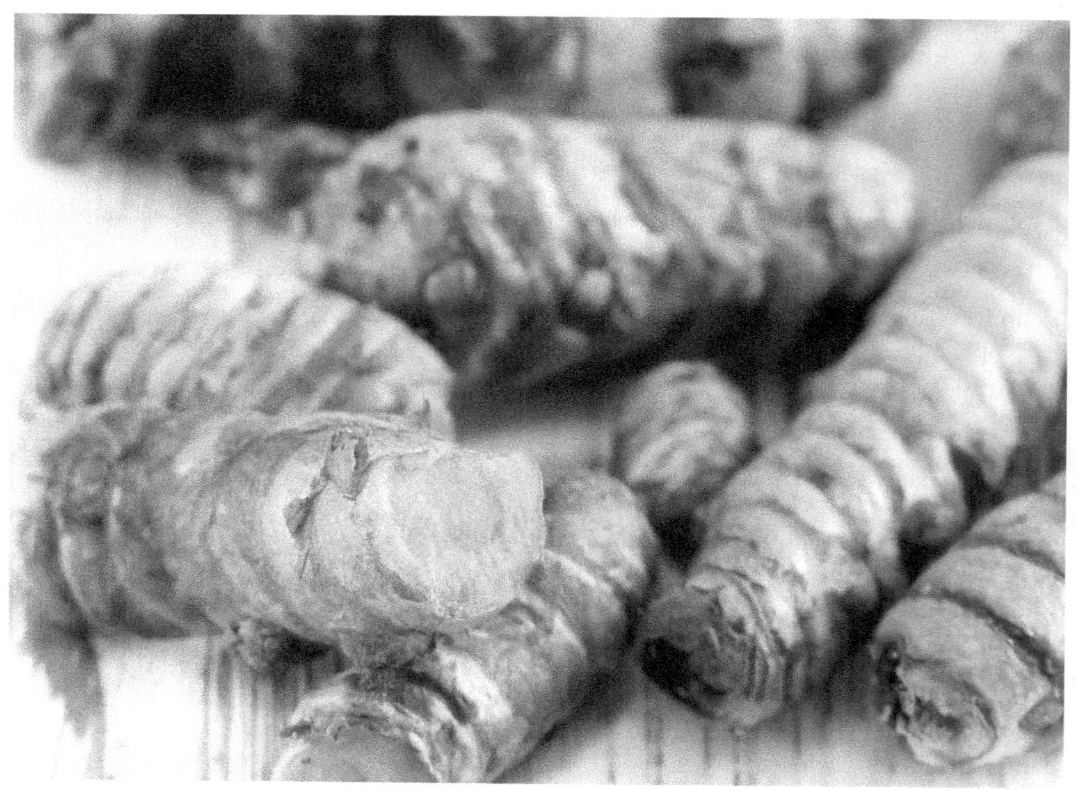

39 TURMERIC

Turmeric is a perennial herbaceous, rhizomatous plant that grows up to 1 meter (3 feet) in height, with dark green leaves, yellowish white flowers, and orange rhizomes, native to Southeast Asia. Turmeric has a long history of use in traditional Chinese medicine, Ayurveda, and Unani.

Common Name(s): Turmeric
Botanical Name(s): *Curcuma longa*
Botanical Family: Zingiberaceaea (ginger family)
Plant Parts Used: Rhizomes (root)
Odor Profile: Earthy pungent
Flavor: Earthy pungent
Safety Considerations: None known.

Biophysical Actions: anti-inflammatory, carminative, rubefacient

Turmeric hydrosol has an earthy, pungent flavor and aroma. It has a slight rubefacient action and is warming, I recommend it for cold, rheumatic joints and muscles that are stagnated and need some warming. Internally, the hydrosol is gently warming, though not as strong as the herb -- but this makes it better received for summer use in hot climates.

Aromatic Chai

4-6 pippali peppers (available at most Indian markets)
6-8 cloves
6-8 allspice berries
2 cinnamon sticks
6 teaspoons rooibos
1 tablespoon dried ginger root (or 2 tablespoons fresh, chopped)
1 tablespoon dried orange peel
4-5 cardamom pods
6 cups filtered water

Place all ingredients in a saucepan, bring to a boil, then simmer, covered, for 20-30 minutes. Strain.

Add:

15-30 mls (1-2 tablespoons) hydrosol(s) – cinnamon, turmeric, tulsi, and/or cardamom
Milk (dairy or non)
Sweetener – honey or maple syrup

Serve warm.

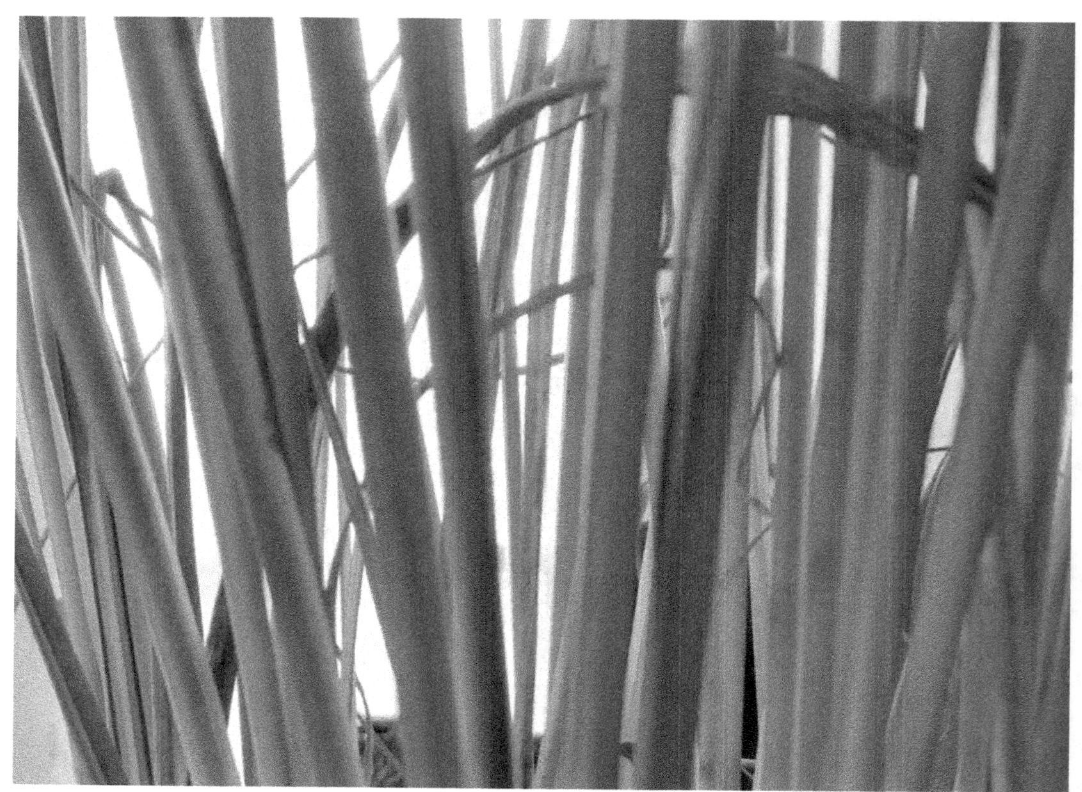

40 VETIVER

Vetiver is a grass native to India that grows up to 1.5 meters (5 feet) in height, with roots that grow downward 2-4 meters (7-13 feet). The grass has stiff, erect leaves and the roots make it an ideal plant for erosion control and drought-tolerant landscaping in temperate climates.

Common Name(s): Vetiver, Khus
Botanical Name(s): *Vetiveria zizanoides, Andropogon zizanoides, Chrysopogon zizanoides, Phalaris zizanoides*
Botanical Family: Poaceae (grass family)
Plant Parts Used: Root
Odor Profile: Earthy
Flavor: Musky, woody, herbaceous and slighty rosey

Safety Considerations: None known.
Biophysical Actions: nervine, sedative

Vetiver is a cooling and grounding hydrosol that suits well to calming the nervous system and dispersing heat. I reach for this hydrosol for insomnia in hot weather, nightsweats, heat rash, and hypertension related to anger and frustration. It can be a powerful relaxant, so beware of using this during the day and then trying to return to mental tasks or drive a vehicle.

Khus Sharbat

A sharbat is an aromatic simple syrup that can be enjoyed as is with a dessert spoon, or diluted in water or milk.

1 cup filtered water
3/4 cup raw sugar
5 mls (1 teaspoon) vetiver (khus) hydrosol

In a small saucepan, heat the water and sugar on medium, until sugar has dissolved and a syrup has formed. Remove from heat and let cool before adding hydrosol. Transfer to a jar and refrigerate until chilled. Can be drizzled over vanilla ice cream, added to a glass of sparkling water or chilled almond milk, or used as a base for chopped seasonal fruit, like strawberries or mango.

Khus Kulfi

Kulfi is a traditional Indian popsicle and I've combined several of my favorite Indian flavors in this recipe.

2 cups milk (whole cow milk is traditional, but coconut milk works nicely here too)
2 teaspoons arrowroot powder
1/4 cup raw sugar
12-15 pistachios, finely chopped in the food processor
1/4 cup heavy cream (or coconut cream)
5 mls (1 teaspoon) Rose hydrosol
5 mls (1 teaspoon) Vetiver hydrosol

In a small bowl, mix arrowroot powder with 1/2 cup milk until smooth, then set aside. Add remaining 1-1/2 cups milk to a medium-sized saucepan and bring to a simmer over medium heat, stirring constantly. Lower heat to medium-low and slowly stir in arrowroot milk, whisking well to prevent lumps from forming. Cook for 5 minutes, stirring constantly. Remove from heat and let cool. Whisk in chopped pistachio pieces, heavy cream, and the hydrosols. Transfer to popsicle molds and freeze overnight.

Glossary of Therapeutic Terms

Analgesic - numbs pain locally.

Anodyne - reduces or relieves pain.

Antibacterial - destructive to bacteria.

Anti-contusion - reduces discoloration and swelling of bruised tissue.

Antifungal - inhibits growth of fungus.

Anti-infectious - helps the body strengthen its own resistance to infectious organisms and rid the body of illness.

Anti-inflammatory - alleviates inflammation.

Antipyretic - dispels heat, fire and fever (from the Greek word *pyre*, meaning fire).

Antiseptic - assists in fighting germs/infections.

Antispasmodic - relieves spasms of voluntary and involuntary muscles.

Antirheumatic - prevents and/or relieves rheumatic pain and swelling.

Antiviral - inhibits growth of viruses.

Anxiolytic - reduces or relieves anxiety or feelings of anxiousness.

Astringent - firms tissue and organs; reduces discharges and secretions.

Carminative - relieves intestinal gas pain and distention; promotes peristalsis.

Cephalic - remedy for the head, usually clearing and stimulating.

Cicatrisant - cell-regenerative for skin, healing for scars.

Decongestant - reduces nasal mucus production and swelling.

Depurative - purifying action.

Diaphoretic - causes perspiration and increased elimination through the skin.

Diuretic - promotes activity of kidney and bladder and increases urination.

Emmenagogue - helps promote and regulate menstruation.

Expectorant - promotes discharge of phlegm and mucus from the lungs and throat.

Hypotensive - lowers high blood pressure.

Immune stimulant - stimulates functioning of the immune system.

Mucolytic - breaks down mucus (pulmonary).

Nervine - strengthens the functional activity of the nervous system; may be either a stimulant or sedative.

Rubefacient - causes an increase in local blood circulation, can causes minor skin irritation, vasodilation and local analgesic effect.

Sedative - calms and tranquilizes by lowering the functional activity of the organ or body part.

Stimulant - increases functional activity of specific organ or system.

Sudorific - increases sweating.

Vasodilator - helps to dilate blood vessels.

References

6th Happiness, curry plant blooming. (2010). Licensed under Creative Commons –Share Alike 3.0 Unported license.

Borgatti, M., et al., (2011). Bergamot (Citrus bergamia Risso) fruit extracts and identified components alter expression of interleukin 8 gene in cystic fibrosis bronchial epithelial cell lines. *BMC biochemistry, 12*(1), p.1.

Bradley, P.R. , (1992). *British Herbal Compendium,* Vol. 1. Bournemouth: British Herbal Medicine Association.

Brakie, M. (2010). Plant fact sheet for American beautyberry (*Callicarpa Americana*). USDA-Natural Resources Conservation Service, East Texas Plant Materials Center.

Buckle, J., (2014). Clinical aromatherapy: Essential oils in practice. Elsevier Health Sciences.

Cosentino M., Luini A., Bombelli R., Corasaniti M. T., Bagetta G., and Marino F. (2014), *The Essential Oil of Bergamot Stimulates Reactive Oxygen Species Production in Human Polymorphonuclear Leukocytes, Phytother. Res., 28, 1232*–1239. doi: 10.1002/ptr.5121.

Day, John and Peta. Fragonia™. (2006). Used with permission from The Paperbark Co.

Decroix, L., Tonoli, C., Soares, D. D., Tagougui, S., Heyman, E., & Meeusen, R. (2016). Acute cocoa flavanol improves cerebral oxygenation without enhancing executive function at rest or after exercise. *Applied Physiology, Nutrition, and Metabolism, 41*(12), 1225-1232.

Faucon, M., (2012). Traité d'aromathépie scientifique et médicale. Sang de la Terre.

Grass, G., Rensing, C., & Solioz, M. (2011). Metallic copper as an antimicrobial surface. Applied and environmental microbiology, 77(5), 1541-1547.

Harman, A. "Hydrolats and Current Research: Chemistry, Microbiology and Stability." Botanica 2012, September 7-10, 2012, Dublin, Ireland, edited by Rhiannon Lewis, International Journal of Clinical Aromatherapy.

Harman, A., (2015). Harvest to Hydrosol: Distill Your Own Exquisite Hydrosols at Home.

Hobbs, C. (1996). Vitex, The Women's Herb. Santa Cruz: Botanica Press.

Holmes, P (2001) Clinical Aromatherapy: Using Essential Oils for Healing Body & Soul. Tiger Lily Press.

References Continued

Iseki, A., Kambe, F., Okumura, K., Hayakawa, T., & Seo, H. (2000). Regulation of Thyroid Follicular Cell Function by Intracellular Redox-Active Copper 1. Endocrinology, 141(12), 4373-4382.

Kreydin, A., (2015) Bergamot Monograph.

Kreydin, A., (2015) Chamomile, Roman Monograph.

Kreydin, A., (2014) Clary Sage Monograph.

Kreydin, A., (2014) Frankincense Monograph.

Kreydin, A., (2015) Geranium Monograph.

Kreydin, A., (2015) Ginger Monograph.

Kreydin, A., (2015) Lavender Monograph.

Kreydin, A., (2016) Lemon Monograph.

Kreydin, A., (2016) Peppermint Monograph.

Kreydin, A., (2016) Rosemary Monograph.

Kreydin, A., (2016) Tea Tree Monograph.

Laitche. *Pelargonium graveolens.* (2008). Public Domain.

Meneerke bloem. *Salvia sclarea.* (2010). Licensed under Creative Commons Attribution-Share Alike 3.0 Unported license.

Mojay, G (1997) *Aromatherapy for Healing the Spirit.* Healing Arts Press.

Oestreicher, P., & Cousins, R. J. (1985). Copper and zinc absorption in the rat: mechanism of mutual antagonism. The Journal of nutrition, 115(2), 159-166.

Peterson C, Rowley W, Coats J. (2001). Catnip Essential Oil as a Mosquito Repellent. American Chemical Society's 222nd National Meeting, 2001 Aug 26-30; Chicago.

Price, L., & Price, S. (2004). Understanding hydrolats: the specific hydrosols for aromatherapy: a guide for health professionals. Churchill Livingstone.

Robinson, C. (2006) A New Essential Oil – Agonis fragrans: Chemotype Selection and Evaluation. Rural Industries Research and Development Corporation.

Rose, J., (2013). The Aromatherapy Book. North Atlantic Books.

References Continued

Schulz, V., R. Hänsel, V.E. Tyler. (1998). Rational Phytotherapy: A Physicians' Guide to Herbal Medicine. New York: Springer.

Sheppard-Hanger S., (1995). The Aromatherapy Practitioner Reference Manual Vol 1 & 2.

Sherwood Taylor, F. (1937). The origins of Greek alchemy. Ambix, 1(1), 30-47.

Singh, N., Verma, P., Pandey, B. R., & Bhalla, M. (2012). Therapeutic potential of Ocimum sanctum in prevention and treatment of cancer and exposure to radiation: An overview. *International Journal of pharmaceutical sciences and drug research*, 4(2), 97-104.

Starr, Forest & Kim. Plants of Hawaii Image 070906-8819. (2007). Licensed under Creative Commons Attribution 3.0 Unported license.
Available: http://www.hear.org/starr/plants/images/image/?q=070906-8819.

Tisserand, Young (2014) Essential Oil Safety 2e. Churchill Livingstone.

Valnet, J (1980, 1990) The Practice of Aromatherapy. Healing Arts Press.

World Health Organization. (2004). *WHO monographs on selected medicinal plants* (Vol. 2). World Health Organization.

Resources

In my private practice I support women and family-owned businesses with a history of providing quality products and having strong relationships with the growers, harvesters, and distillers/producers. Please refer to the questions in *What to Look for in a Quality Hydrosol* chapter to help guide you as you choose companies to purchase quality hydrosols from. Here are some companies I have had the pleasure of sampling hydrosols from:

Aromaceuticals, owned by aromatherapist Katharine Koeppen in California, carries a small selection of hydrolats (hydrosols). http://aromaceuticals.com.

Morning Myst Botanics, formerly owned by Ann Harman, this artisan distillation company specializes in producing hydrosols, not biowaste. They have a nice selection of hydrosols starting at 1 gallon volume. http://morningmystbotanics.com.

Mountain Rose Herbs, owned by herbalist Julie Bailey, carries a moderate selection of hydrosols. http://mountainroseherbs.com.

Nature's Gift, owned by Marge Clark in Tennessee, carries a nice selection of hydrosols. http://naturesgift.com.

Snow Lotus, owned by aromatherapist Peter Holmes, carries a small selection of hydrosols. http://snowlotus.org.

StillPoint Aromatics, owned by aromatherapists Joy Musacchio and Cynthia Brownley in Arizona, carries a nice selection of hydrosols. http://stillpointaromatics.com.

SunRose Aromatics, owned by Roseanne Tarturo in Maine, carries a moderate selection of hydrosols. http://sunrosearomatics.com.

Facebook Groups

Facebook groups I can recommend on hydrosols are:

Artisan Essential Oil Distillers, a large group headed by American perfumist Jessica Ring, from Oregon. Not exclusive to essential oils, many hydrosol distillers are in this group too. https://www.facebook.com/groups/1397983977111787.

"Hydrosols" – Herbs&Aromatherapy, led by beloved aromatherapy educator Jeanne Rose, from California. Ms Rose is the author of several books on aromatherapy. https://www.facebook.com/groups/hydrosols.

Aromatic Waters: Hydrosols, a group for this book! Come discuss recipes, experiences, and your favorite hydrosols. https://www.facebook.com/groups/aromaticwaters

Resources Continued

Aromaweb.com, informational website with profiles on hydrosols and general information on aromatherapy by Wendy Robbins.
http://aromaweb.com

The Barefoot Dragonfly, offering an Aromatic Waters companion e-course, and other educational resources on hydrosols.
http://thebarefootdragonfly.com/learning-center/aromatic-waters/

Circle H Institute, an online resource from distiller and author Ann Harman. Membership provides access to reports on microbiological testing of dozens of hydrosols, GCMS lab testing on over a hundred hydrosols, and abstract titles of research papers on hydrosols.
https://circlehinstitute.com

Books

Many of the hydrosol books on the market are over a decade old and in desperate need of updating with more modern practices, new research, and data that has accrued over the past 10-15 years. Keeping that in mind it is quite possible to still find useful data in some of the older books when compared side-by-side with research papers and testing data.

Harvest to Hydrosol: Distill Your Own Exquisite Hydrosols at Home (2015), by Ann Harman – a modern resource for those looking for guidance on the process of distilling hydrosols.

Understanding Hydrolats: The Specific Hydrosols for Aromatherapy (2004), by Len Price and Shirley Price – used in conjunction with more modern testing of hydrosols this book is a helpful resource for therapeutic dosing.

Hydrosols: The Next Aromatherapy (2001), by Suzanne Catty – used in conjunction with more modern testing of hydrosols you may find some creative ideas for formulating with hydrosols in this book.

Acknowledgements

I am very grateful to my students and clients who have peppered me with questions, trusted me to be part of their wellness teams, and otherwise given me the opportunity to write a book based on these experiences.

A big thank you to my proofreaders/editors: Ann Gordon, Tess Clark, and Brandi Blaisdell. This team helped me polish this book into a readable format; fixing spelling mistakes, correcting punctuation, and reminding me of the book's audience. Thank you, ladies!

Thank you to my husband, Oleg, who has supported me in all of my Barefoot Dragonfly endeavors over the years, including this project. For your tireless cheerleading, reminders for me to eat when I get lost in writing and research, and being my 'math guy' when I need help sorting out a formula, thank you. This book could not have happened without you, Babe!

Thank you to my parents, who nurtured my love of plants and wellness from a young age, and who have been willing test subjects for a myriad aromatic remedies. A special thanks to my mother who braved bear season with me during my first foray into wildcrafting for hydrosols so we could collect Pinyon and Ponderosa pine needles at 9,000 feet in elevation.

Thank you to the aromatherapy community who has shaped me into the aromatherapist I am today. Your support, companionship, and dance parties have enriched my career and personal life in more ways than I can enumerate. A special thanks to my teachers and mentors, Kathy Duffy, Sylla Sheppard-Hangar, Robert Tisserand, Mark Webb, Peter Holmes, Gabriel Mojay, Jeanne Rose, Marco Valusi, Jack Chaitman, Ann Harman, Marge Clark, and Rhiannon Lewis.

Thank you, reader, for supporting me through the purchase of this book; I hope you've found new ways to use hydrosols in your wellness plan.

www.ingramcontent.com/pod-product-compliance
Lightning Source LLC
Chambersburg PA
CBHW080854260726
48660CB00009B/3302